THE

PARADIGM

DIET

~

Principles of Proper Nutrition

ADAM DAVE, M.D.

Cover design: Kerstin John
www.kerstinjohn.com

To Mom and Dad, for showing the way.

And

To Kerstin, for walking with me.

CONTENTS

PARADIGM PRAISE

"*The Paradigm Diet* is an excellent guide on how to put a plant-based diet to work for your health. Whether it's to slim down or increase energy, this guide will help you get there."

　　- Neal Barnard, M.D., President, Physicians Committee for Responsible Medicine

"Dr. Dave joins the battle against common dietary disease with *The Paradigm Diet*. This is a worthwhile read in your effort to regain [and maintain] your health and appearance."

　　- John McDougall, M.D., Author and Founder of the McDougall Program

"*The Paradigm Diet* offers an approach to food that's both time-honored and backed by scientific evidence. With wit and eloquence, Dr. Dave makes complex medical concepts mainstream. After you read this book, you'll know more about nutrition than many doctors and be able to cook healthier meals than most 5-star chefs."

　　- Harvey Diamond, Best-selling Author of *Fit for Life*

"*The Paradigm Diet* is the best book I have read about nutrition and exercise (and the ethical life of food choices). It provides more useful information about diet than any book on the topic, much more than a 'med school's worth'."

　　- Danny Burns, M.D., Ph.D., Professor, Anatomical Sciences, Assistant Dean of Students, St. George's School of Medicine

"*The Paradigm Diet* has so much good information."

    - Joel Fuhrman, M.D., Best-selling Author of *Eat to Live*

"Adam Dave, M.D. helps us live a healthy lifestyle with his simple, straight-forward message about diet and exercise."

    - Elson M. Haas, M.D., Integrated Medicine Practitioner and Author of *Staying Healthy with Nutrition*

"*The Paradigm Diet* strikes a delicate balance between providing adequate scientific information and a practical approach to healthy dietary habits."

    - Abboud J. Ghalayini, Ph.D., Professor, Department of Biochemistry, St. George's University School of Medicine

"After just a few weeks I have lost a whole pants size and my cholesterol dropped over 100 points. I feel more confident and energetic. Plus, this *dietstyle* has trickled down to my wife and son."

    - Justin Bauer, Mensa Vice President, Inland Empire

"I like the vegetables, the fruits, the beans, the stuff I eat now."

    - Former U.S. President Bill Clinton, who has lost over 20 lbs on a vegan diet

HORS D'OEUVRE

Dear Friend,

Health is more than merely the absence of disease. It is vitality, wholeness and harmony of the body, mind and soul.

The food you eat transforms itself into the cells that shape your body, power your heart, transmit brain waves and modulate your mood. As diet influences how we look, think and feel, it is truly the doorway to health.

Proper nutrition is only one component of a healthy lifestyle, but it may be the most important. Without adequate nourishment, the other areas of life are thrown out of whack and the individual is bound to suffer.

A toxic diet deprives the body of nutrients and fills it with empty calories and harmful chemicals. This constipates the cells, deranges the blood sugar and saturates the bloodstream with acids and fats. Fatigue results, and physical activity becomes difficult and unpleasant.

As movement diminishes, depression sets in and with it the symptoms of restlessness and distractibility. An overfed, undernourished, sedentary body slows the mind and blunts the emotions, and the soul starves as relationships and artistic expression suffer. Sadness, loss of interest in daily activities, weight gain, difficulty sleeping and feelings of worthlessness fill up one's days. Suicide, or thoughts of it, may be the unfortunate consequence.

Contrast this to what one feels from eating nutritiously. From wise culinary choices flows improved energy leading to increased physical activity, which sharpens mental clarity, elevates consciousness, even enhances your capacity to feel.

Harmony of body, mind and soul, starting with good food.

Diet is the doorway to this harmony, and you hold the key.

The purpose of this book is threefold.

First, to *provide* you with the principles of proper nutrition.

Next, to *prove* beyond any doubt the healthiest diet on the planet.

Finally, to *propose* a practical means of implementing this diet that is easy, efficient, affordable and fun for one and all.

The Paradigm Diet is easy to digest, pardon the pun. Read it with enjoyment and care, so that you may incorporate its principles at once - at the market, in the kitchen and at your next meal - to nourish yourself and those you love, with results that are both rapid and permanent.

WHO SHOULD READ THIS BOOK

Let's face it, as a race, we humans have forgotten how to eat, and as individuals, most of us never even learned. We unconsciously stuff ourselves with high-fat animal products and refined empty calories and then marvel as over time our bodies get heavier and the list of aches, pains and other ailments grows longer.

You may say, *Not me! My diet is pretty good, and I'm not as heavy as some people I know.*

It sounds like you need a little convincing. Let's take a look in the mirror and see what we see, shall we?

We can start with the top 13 food sources of calories among Americans ages 2 and older.

donuts

bread

chicken

pizza

pasta

burritos

beef

ice cream

potato chips

burgers

milk

cheese

cereal[1]

What do all 13 have in common - other than being delicious, you might say? They are without exception, either refined, processed carbs or high-fat animal protein.

The result of this diet?

Thirty-four percent of the population is obese.

Over 80 million Americans – over one third of the population – have heart disease.

Nearly half of us have or are at risk of having diabetes.

Seventy percent have or are in danger of developing high blood pressure.

And almost 1 in 2 Americans will be diagnosed with cancer during your lifetime. Notice how we said *your*. That's either you or your spouse. Maybe both.

Okay, now you may be saying, *I'm not one of these people. I'm me. And I eat healthy!*

Though you may think so, chances are that if you consumed a packaged food item within the last 24 hours, whether you bought it at a health food store or a gas station, that food contains refined carbohydrate, high fat animal products, or both. And both are junk. So you see, even if you don't patronize McDonald's, your diet can still use a makeover.

Who else? As was said in *Top Gun*: The list is long, but distinguished.[2]

If you suffer from low energy, this book is for you.

If your nights are filled with pizza and your days spent in a junk food haze, this book is for you.

If your days are spent in a junk food haze and your nights are spent dreaming of pizza, this book is for you.

If you get tired after lunch and wish you could take a nap, this book is for you.

If you can't sleep at night, this book is for you.

If you fall asleep in class or at work, this book is for you. If you fell asleep in health class, are currently enrolled in health class, loved health class and learned everything, or hate learning and are sleeping as you read this, this book is for you.

If you are a nurse, nutritionist, medical student or doctor, this book is for you.

If you think acetyl-CoA is a clothing line or type of gasoline, this book is for you.

If your desire is to develop a working knowledge of nutrition, this book is for you.

If you have ever asked yourself or someone else where you get your protein, this book is for you.

If you think milk is a good source of calcium, this book is for you.

If you think fish is a health food, this book is for you.

If you think whole grains or nuts are wholesome and nutritious and gobble down bread by the loaf and peanuts by the handful, this book is for you.

If you don't like vegetables, this book is for you.

If you love vegetables but don't know how to prepare them, this book is for you.

If you don't eat enough fiber, this book is for you. If you think you eat enough fiber, this book is for you.

If your medicine cabinet contains more than a multivitamin, this book is for you.

If you think it is bad to eat a big meal before bed, this book is for you.

If you are a vegan, this book is for you. If you think vegans are self-righteous prigs, this book is for you.

If you think soy products are your friends, this book is for you.

If you think it's a bad idea to eat late at night, this book is for you.

If you hate to cook, this book is for you.

If you love to cook, this book is for you.

If you think it's important to drink tons of water, this book is for you.

If you love to eat and hate to restrict yourself to palm-sized portions of your favorite foods to keep your weight in check, this book is for you.

If you are obsessed with food, binge eat from time to time, are constantly plagued by food cravings, or feel guilty after eating, this book is for you.

If you believe you know everything there is to know about nutrition and your diet is perfect, this book is for you.

If you could stand to shed a few pounds, this book is for you.

If you could stand to shed more than a few pounds, this book is for you.

If you believe you're at the perfect weight, this book is for you.

If you wish to gain weight and think the only way to "bulk up" is by eating a lot of animal protein, boy do we have news for you.

If you want to find out what doctors learn in medical school without getting lost in confusing concepts and terms, this book is for you.

If you want to know more about nutrition than most doctors and be able to cook healthier food than many 5-star chefs, this book is for you.

Let's see, are we leaving anyone out? Oh, yes: YOU!

So start reading *The Paradigm Diet* now and read it cover to cover. Don't skip or skim. Whether it takes you one afternoon or an entire year, take it all in.

Some of the topics presented here will challenge what you hold as sacred and true. To wit:

It's bad to eat late at night. (False!)

Eat several small meals throughout the day. (False!)

Drink lots of water. (False!)

Milk gives you strong bones. (False!)

Animal foods (meat, eggs, dairy) are highest in protein. (False!)

Olive oil is good for you. (False!)

Nuts are healthy fats. (False!)

Fruit is high in sugar. (False!)

A healthy diet should include several servings per day of whole grains. (You guessed it: False!)

As these and other popular myths come crumbling before your eyes, you may feel shocked and shaken to the core.

Then, as you eat larger quantities of food than you ever imagined, you'll feel satisfied, and relieved.

Finally, as you experience more energy and weigh less than ever before in your adult life, you'll never be the same.

And you'll find that you quite like the change.

So, join us on the journey. Kiss the past goodbye, and welcome the New You!

Remember, food is meant to delight your taste buds and to nourish your body. If it fails to do either of these, it has failed you. If you have an antagonistic relationship with food, craving what is high in calories and low in nutrition, binging on empty calories and then feeling racked with shame, you are the victim.

A solid footing in the culinary art will make you immune to untruth. By gaining an intimate familiarity with the principles of proper nutrition, by learning the language of gastronomy, you can empower yourself to make nutritious, delicious food choices at each and every meal. Only by arming yourself with a sound knowledge of digestive anatomy and physiology can you win the war on your health and the fight for your life. And frankly, this is exactly what's at stake.

Why be slave to your urges and preyed upon by advertisers and food chemists and big corporations when you can take charge of your diet and life?

It's time that you become the Master.

A bit about me: I grew up in Los Angeles, the eldest of three boys. Mom and dad raised us as vegetarians, which was and still is an all-too-rare occurrence. However, eggs and dairy products did feature prominently at our family's table. In college I took up weight-lifting, going every afternoon to Gold's Gym, Venice, also known as the Mecca of Bodybuilding. Convinced by friends that I needed to eat meat to get big and strong, I began to include animal products in my diet. First it was turkey sandwiches to supplement egg white omelettes and protein shakes. Then came the steaks. Big, juicy steaks. Soon I was eating whole chickens for dinner! I kid you not. It was called the Bodybuilder's Dinner and featured an entire chicken, skinless and roasted.

On this regimen, I got strong. Boy did I ever. Soon I was bench-pressing nearly 300 lbs. And I also gained weight. In about 3 months, I went from 165 lbs (my high school graduation weight) to 190 lbs. But along with the increase in size and strength came other characteristics that were, well, not so pleasant. These included a terrible case of acne that ran the length of my neck and included in its trail my back and shoulders; fits of poor energy that made it impossible some mornings to drag myself out of bed in time for class; and I also suffered severe mood swings, prompting friends (the same friends who recommended I eat meat) to suspect I was taking steroids. But I wasn't! Oh, but I was. (Animal protein contains estrogen and testosterone.)

Clearly the transformation my body and personality had undergone were the direct results of my dietary modifications, specifically eating meat, as nothing else in my life had changed during this time. I didn't know it back then, but I had successfully conducted an experiment on the effects of meat consumption – an *experiment of one*, if you will. Overnight I had gone from eating no meat to eating lots of meat, and I wore the results in my big muscles and on my pock-marked face. The scars would eventually fade, as would my meat-centric diet. But the experiments continued.

In the years that led up to medical school, I experimented with a variety of approaches to food, including juice fasts and "low-carb" diets. On these and other fads I would experience the same results. I would lose weight quickly, only to quickly gain it back, which is what happens to most people following this approach, maybe even you. Convinced that my protein requirements could only be met by consuming some animal products, I never gave veganism a try, even though it seemed intuitive that plant foods are better for us than animal foods. I sensed my knowledge of nutrition was lacking, so I enrolled in medical school, which, I would come to learn, is the last place to look for nutritional advice. A paltry two textbook chapters in four years of medical education!

After graduating, I entered family medicine and trained as a resident physician in a nationally-ranked, university-based teaching hospital. Indeed the University of Colorado offers a fine training program in general medicine – with one exception. You guessed it: nutrition. On my first day of residency, I was told that lifestyle factors – specifically diet, exercise, smoking, drinking and bodyweight – account for 85 percent of all disease. I was urged to counsel patients on smoking cessation and to advise that patients drink in moderation and get enough exercise. But when it came to diet, all I could offer was a blank stare. I was learning loads about medications, procedures, diseases and their treatments, but nothing about prevention through food! And so when asked by patients for dietary advice, I'd simply refer to a dietician or abashedly mumble something about the USDA food pyramid, which as we shall see is, in many respects, an example of what NOT to do.

What medicine did instil, if not an understanding of nutritional science, were the research and analytical skills to weed through pseudoscience (the territory of fads and false claims) and focus on the facts: solid, scientifically-based facts. My medical training familiarized me with reputable sources to whom (and to which) to turn to receive scientifically-sound information.

And what I learned astounded me, both for its simplicity and its practicability. No supplements, no fancy methods of preparation, no counting calories. No monitoring portion sizes or worrying about specific nutrients. Just good clean food.

In the pages that follow, I am proud to provide you with the course on nutrition that doctors should be taught, indeed that everyone should learn, and then you'll be able to apply this knowledge for yourself.

THE PARADIGM PROMISE

By simply changing your approach to food, you can do all this and more:

1. Lose 15 lbs or more, in just 3 weeks![3]

2. Eat as much as you want and still lose weight.[4]

3. Increase your metabolism, naturally.[5]

4. Cut your cholesterol in half, without medication![6]

5. Drastically reduce your risk of diabetes, cancer and other diet-related illnesses. If you are diabetic, reduce your insulin requirements, and possibly discontinue medication altogether.[7]

6. Greatly reduce your risk of high blood pressure. If you have hypertension, lower your blood pressure naturally, without medication.[8]

7. Improve your memory.[9]

8. Prevent and reverse heart disease, without invasive procedures or expensive medication.

9. Live longer.[10]

10. Be stronger and faster, without working out.[11]

Dear Parents:

In an age of abundance, we live in a world of famine.

We feast on calorie-dense, nutrient-poor foods that are genetically modified, mass-produced, chemically-engineered and prepared by strangers to seduce our taste buds while they starve our cells. These empty calories - an increasing number of which are **disguised as health foods** - leave us overfed and undernourished. They encourage over-indulgence and give rise to constant cravings, obesity and a host of other maladies. This happens in every neighborhood throughout the world, every day at every meal. It is likely occurring to some degree even in your own home.

The average person's diet consists mainly of refined, processed carbohydrates and high-fat animal protein. Over 90 percent of what we eat is of little nutritional value. In other words, it is junk. Most people eat way too many calories (over 3,500 calories per day[12]), too much meat and dairy (more than two lbs per day[13]) and far too little produce. In fact, less than 15 percent of Americans consume the recommended 5 daily servings of fruits and vegetables, and even for those that do, produce makes up a mere 10 percent of total caloric intake.[14]

And for many kids, syrupy fruit drinks make up most of their fruit intake and half of their vegetable consumption is in the form of French fries, a food so devoid of nutrition that many health experts do not even consider it a vegetable![15]

Meat products, on the other hand, are devoured in superabundance. Over a lifetime, the standard American diet provides each person with 2,000 chickens, 7 cattle and 12 pigs, eaten through and through. That's a lot of flesh!

The take-home message is this: Your diet is very likely in need of a serious make-over.

If you make a conscious effort to eat nutritious foods, shop at health-food stores and load up on supplements, your diet is more than likely deficient in one or more major nutrients. So-called health foods such as deli salads often come drenched in oil. Supplements such as energy bars, meal replacement drinks and protein powders contain a mishmash of highly-concentrated, heavily-processed ingredients that spells disaster for the digestion. And though pills may provide large doses of a few vitamins and minerals, they fail to match the cornucopia of nutrients present in whole foods.

Even if you are a vegan, your nutritional status is likely bordering on red. Yes, a plant-based diet is the healthiest on the planet, we'll allow. (How's that for putting our cards on the table!) But too many vegans lull themselves into complacency with expensive, over-processed soy products and an over-reliance on grains. They fail to consume sufficient quantities of whole foods, specifically fruits and vegetables, the result of which includes anemia, fatigue, constipation, bloat and gas. Foul-smelling, fetid flatulence. Lingering farts! There, we said it.

The results of the dietary fiasco that is sweeping America and most of the developed world are not only stinky, they are dangerous and can even be deadly. Childhood obesity is at an all-time high and increasing. This sets the stage for chronic illnesses including heart disease, diabetes and high blood pressure. Poor food choices are associated with early puberty, which has been linked to reproductive cancers.

While a poor diet causes disease and hastens death, proper nutrition strengthens the immune system, prevents illness and reverses aging. In fact, the childhood diet is perhaps the greatest predictor of one's health later in life. If it is so important, why is it so often ignored?

Efforts to improve school nutrition do exist; however, they are largely misguided. Certain foods (meat and milk, for instance) still appear in every cafeteria meal despite the overwhelming scientific evidence that they are disease-producing. Despite good intentions, these efforts ultimately fail because they ignore the central truth that nutrition starts in the home. Kids eat what they see their parents eat. And parents eat crap. You'd think the *p* in *parent* stood for pizza, popcorn and potato chips. Jeez! We don't even feed our pets this junk, yet we devour prodigious amounts of these and other processed foods with insatiable relish.

Eating right would be much easier if proper nutrition were taught in school, but it's not. Classroom nutrition is based on the USDA food pyramid, which is loaded with bad advice. Among other things, it allows for the consumption of genetically-modified oils (canola) and empty-calorie foods such as refined grains; it ignores leafy green vegetables and instead recommends milk products as the calcium source though milk can in fact deplete calcium and weaken bones; and it encourages an intake of excessive amounts of fat.

For example, a 13-year-old girl following government guidelines could consume 10 times as much meat and cheese as vegetables. In one day, she could devour 15 egg yolks and 9 slices of processed cheese.[16] That's over 110 grams of fat and over 3,000 mg of cholesterol, 10 times the daily limit. In one day! And we haven't even discussed the crackers, pretzels and white bread she'll be eating in accordance with this diet. The USDA would call her "healthy." If such a manner of eating were kept up, we're afraid her friends would soon be calling her "hefty."

Not versed in the principles of sound nutrition, parents fall prey to fads and false claims. Lacking time, it is tempting to reach for whatever packaged, processed food is at hand and pop it in the microwave, or just order take-out. And while pizza, burgers and fries may please your palate, they most definitely poison your body and drain your expense account. Families who consume most of their meals outside the home typically spend 40 percent more on food than those who prepare their own meals. This can amount to $150 per week, or $7,500 per year, the cost of two years of city college! So, you can *save* up for your family's future and *stave* off the diseases that threaten your future by preparing your own healthy meals. In short, it has never been more important to learn the science of practical nutrition and apply it in your home.

Parents, it is up to you. Your family's life is in your hands.

In fact, it is likely that within the next 35 years (around 2045), Earth's population will have swelled to 10 billion people. To fill all these stomachs, estimates are that global food production will have to double. In the setting of climate change and a finite amount of arable land and drinkable water, a dietary adjustment is crucial, or worldwide famine is inevitable.

It is high time we emphasize foods (fruits, vegetables) that provide more calories per acre, while reducing production of foods like grains that are diverted to animal feed, and eliminating consumption of animal food altogether.

As a family medicine resident at the University of Colorado, patients would often ask me for advice on diet. The "askers" were among a varied group that suffered from one or more of the following: overweight or obesity, high blood pressure, elevated cholesterol, diabetes, autoimmune conditions, in addition to heart disease, cancer and strokes, not to mention less serious ills including acne, urinary tract infections, sinus problems, constipation, irritable bowel, allergies, fatigue, fibromyalgia and chronic pain. Because the study of nutrition is so sorely absent from the standard medical education both in medical school and in residency, I had precious little knowledge about what constitutes the ideal diet, nor was I aware that such a diet is a veritable cure-all for all of the above conditions and more. It was not until I embarked on an independent study of nutrition that my views about food underwent a paradigm shift. It was then that I learned and embraced the Paradigm Diet, which is both time-honored and backed by the latest scientific research.

The leading medical experts are now in agreement that a whole foods, plant-based diet is the healthiest diet on the planet, more effective than medication in the treatment and prevention of a variety of ills. In reality, good food IS medicine. Though they may differ in the particulars - for example, while some recommend nuts and oils, others discourage these foods in favor whole grains - the recommendations made by a growing number of scientists (including Joel Fuhrman, M.D., Dean Ornish, M.D., Neal Barnard, M.D., John McDougall, M.D., T. Colin Campbell, Ph.D., as well as many others) meet in three basic groups: fruits, vegetables and legumes.

Or as we call them, **sweets, greens** and **beans,** in addition to a modest amount of **seeds**.

Despite this agreement, many books on plant-based nutrition encourage consuming large quantities of grains, in addition to loads of processed soy, nuts and even oils. These foods make healthy alternatives to animal foods such as meat and diary, but as we shall see they are *by no means* health foods, and diets centered around grains and nuts can lead to weight gain and other health problems. And yet most vegan or vegetarian diets are much heavier on grains, nuts, oils and soy than they are on fruits, vegetables and beans, when in fact these latter foods are to be the focus of the perfect diet.

In fact, when choosing these foods, you can eat unlimited quantities, because their chemical nature makes them virtually impossible to overeat. Eat as much as you want? No guilt or shame? Food as medicine? Food as *delicious* medicine, with no side effects but excellent health? That's a food lover's dream!

Let's make it yours.

In short, health - not just your own and that of your family, but the health of the entire planet - depends on what YOU eat at each and every meal.

Wow, talk about pressure!

In seriousness, a fast-paced society doesn't have to be a fast-food society. A suffering economy provides the opportunity to return to the basics and find health in simplicity.

You may feel as if you do not have the time or the energy to make lasting improvements in your family's food choices. You may be overworked and overwhelmed. Read this book with your children. Involve them, so that they may take an active role in their health.

In the short time it takes you to peruse these pages, you will learn how to apply the principles of practical nutrition quickly, easily and economically, to make good food a family affair.

And in doing so, you might just save the world.

Kids:

I don't know you, and you may not know this, but chances are you will get cancer or suffer a heart attack, or both, and then you will die.[17]

This is a bummer, and it gets worse: It will probably happen to most of your friends and family, too.

What do these diseases have in common, besides being the biggest killers in our society? They are caused by food. By eating food that has too many calories, not enough nutrients, or both, we make ourselves sick, and then we die. Whoever said "Life is slow suicide" was pretty much right on.

But if you are killing yourself, you are not to blame. It's your mommy and daddy's fault. Just kidding. It's the government's fault. Well, maybe. Fast food should take the blame. In part, yes. But whoever's fault it is, the result is the same:

A fat ass.

Or, if you prefer, junk in your trunk.

Either from bad advice or from sheer ignorance, most kids go off into the world eating whatever is served and serving whatever is easy, and then you grow up to give birth to kids whom you raise much the same way. Bad habits, just like your waist size, and hips, and thighs, and uh, you get the point, have a way of spreading over time, especially when what is involved is food that is cheap and tastes good.

Don't get us wrong. Food should be inexpensive and delicious. But if you care more about how your food tastes and know less about what is in it, you set yourself up for trouble. Ignorance is not bliss. It does not make you happy. Where food is concerned, playing dumb only gets you more junk in the trunk. And who wants junk?

Eating junk food is just as bad for your health as chain smoking and chugging forties. It's frowned upon to smoke and drink in school or at work, is it not? But why is it okay to munch on that greasy steak sandwich right in front of everyone? Why is it okay for cafeterias to serve students and employees fast food? For burger joints, pizzerias and food trucks to be on every street corner? And for vending machines filled with sweet nothings (empty calories) to be available in every hallway, lot and lobby? What gives?

You do.

You pay good money for candies, cookies and other sweet nothings, and here is what you get:

Fatty plaques.

Fatty plaques, or "streaks," as they are also called, are the stuff that builds up on the insides of your blood vessels. These streaks are the first sign of heart disease, and nowadays they are present in the arteries of most teenagers. One hundred years ago heart disease was practically nonexistent, even in adults. Now kids are getting it! So when you are, say, 60 years old and you have your first heart attack, you'll know why: For the last fifty years you clogged your blood with fat and fast food. Don't say we didn't warn you. But you gotta admit, it makes sense. You eat junk, and what you get is just that: junk. Health problems no longer wait for you to grow up. Fast times, these.

Let's leave disease aside and talk about your looks. Like most people, you probably take pride in your appearance (even if you don't want anybody knowing it). And as most know, how you look is a function of how much you weigh. Judging by the numbers, the situation is, well, not pretty. Today, one in three kids has a weight problem. And large kids become really large (obese) adults and then develop chronic conditions that take their money and make their lives miserable, and then they die.

Okay, we're being a bit bleak, but you get the message.

On another note: Maybe you're not worried about your weight and right now you don't really care whether you get sick in twenty or fifty years. Sorry, but you're still not off the hook. Bad food also causes a group of conditions, which though not deadly or disfiguring, can make life a real bitch! These little peskies include allergies, asthma, autoimmune dysfunction, bloating, bad breath, a beer belly, congestion, constipation, dry skin, diarrhea, dark circles, gas, headaches, heart burn, hemorrhoids, irritability, mucus, puffy eyes, stomach cramps, sexual dysfunction, varicose veins and wrinkles. Food can cause alopecia (hair loss) and gynecomastia ("big breasts") in boys, and give girls comedones (zits) and cellulite, or "cottage cheese thighs," as it's also called.

That's right, girls. Cottage cheese. You truly are what you eat.

Luckily, the cause is also the cure. Though bad food can make you sick and tired, good food shoots your energy through the roof. If your goal is to ace the exam, kick butt on the playing field, clear up your skin or trim down for prom, the prescription is, once again, diet. Not any diet, but the perfect diet.

So, what is the perfect diet?

First, we're going to teach you a thing or two about food, but we promise to make it very enjoyable and not the least bit painful. If you are impatient and simply cannot wait to know the Paradigm foods, here is a hint.

Four words.

Sweets. Greens. Beans. Seeds.

That is all.

It's as simple as one, two, three…and one to grow strong and sexy on.

THE PARADIGM DEFINED

par-a-digm [**par**-uh-daym]: an outstandingly clear model

    synonyms: *standard, ideal, paragon, archetype, touchstone*

    broadly: a philosophical or theoretical framework

    example: a *paradigm shift* refers to a change in the way that reality is perceived

Humans are considered omnivores in that we can eat almost anything and survive. Each day, most choose foods from all major food groups, which are **grains**, **dairy**, **protein foods** (meat, poultry and fish, for example), **fruits** and **vegetables**. This seems like a bit of everything. And yet, despite this omnivorous diet, people are getting heavier and sicker than ever. Nearly 70 percent of Americans are overweight or obese. That's more than 2 in 3. The Centers for Disease Control and Prevention estimates that roughly 1 out of 2 people suffers from at least 1 chronic disease, including high blood pressure, heart disease, diabetes and cancer. Though human life expectancy is at an all-time high of 78 years, 1 in 5 persons will die in the Intensive Care Unit, with an average stay of 13 days, and a cost of roughly $25,000. The average cost of a funeral is over $7,000.

This sounds more like suffering than surviving, let alone thriving! Besides, we can think of a lot of ways to spend over 30 grand that are much more fun than a death certificate and a coffin.

Which begs the question: Are we indeed omnivores?

To be well - to thrive - means eating the food we are designed to eat. This food is simple, and it's the same for us all.

Everyone agrees that humans need air - oxygen - to breathe. Imagine if some so-called expert came along and said that because of variations in lungs, no single type of oxygen is suitable for everybody. That person would be laughed off the planet, wouldn't they? And yet, you hear it all the time that based on blood type, or body type, or cravings, or lifestyle, or genetics, or metabolism, there are different diets for different people.

This is baloney.

To take the lung analogy a bit further, there are really only two types of air: clean air and polluted air, with degrees of pollution depending on things such as cars, factories, green plants, wind currents, and so on. It is the same with food. There is food that nourishes the cells, and food that pollutes them. The food that nourishes is the perfect food in that it exactly fits its purpose; other foods are merely degrees of food pollution, some bad, some worse.

Though the ideal diet should focus exclusively on the most nutritious food, it should also be, among other things, easy on your wallet and out-of-this-world delicious too.

It would seem that for a food to be considered ideal, or Paradigm, it should be <u>maximally nutritious</u>, <u>innately delicious</u>, <u>available and affordable</u>, <u>properly prepared</u>, <u>environmentally friendly</u>, <u>unrefined, unprocessed and whole</u>.

Maximally nutritious

As far as one's health is concerned, of these characteristics by far the most important is maximal nutrition, which is a function of nutrient content per calorie. It is simple. The more nutrients in a particular food, the greater its nutritiousness.

Innately delicious

Deliciousness without nutritiousness encourages overindulgence, metabolic derangements and weight gain. Deliciousness by way of chemicals and artificial flavors is designed to deceive our taste buds and cause us to eat what we would otherwise avoid. This is not natural, it is deception. Only food that is both wholesome **and** innately, or naturally, tasty best supports and promotes health and deserves to be called **Paradigm**.

Available and affordable

If a food is nutritious and delicious yet exotic or cost-prohibitive, it is as useful to the empty stomach as thin air. The perfect food is modestly priced and available at the local market, so that it may be a regular feature of the diet.

Properly prepared

And if a food is nutritious, delicious, available and affordable, yet cooked in a way that depletes or deranges its nutrients and replaces them with toxic fats, what remains are empty calories that offer no benefit and may actually cause harm. Improperly prepared foods can easily become disease-promoting rather than life-sustaining.

Take cooking with oil, for example. Heating oil deranges the fats and creates carcinogens. These substances can cause cancer. We don't want that, do we?

The ideal, or Paradigm, food must be prepared in such a way that **preserves or enhances** both taste and nutrition. Fortunately, the healthiest methods of preparing food are without exception the easiest and quickest.

Environmentally friendly

Though a particular food may nourish the individual and possess all of the above characteristics, if it is toxic to the environment or increases pain and suffering in any way, then it is of greater harm than good and cannot be considered ideal. In fact, it would be better if such a food never existed in the first place.

In order to be called Paradigm, a food should require a relative minimum of resources and regenerate rather than ravage the environment, while being a source of pleasure and life rather than pain and death.

Unrefined, unprocessed and whole

And finally, it is not enough to take the thirty or so essential vitamins and minerals, jumble them together and package them in a pill or powder. Nutrition is a relatively young science. There are thousands of nutrients that have not yet been discovered, and supplements do not contain nutrients in the same ratios that exist in nature. (For example, vitamin A in the diet may prevent cancer, but if taken as beta-carotene in supplement form it can increase cancer's incidence. You see, too much of one type of vitamin - in this case carotenoids - may hinder the activity of others.)

The ideal or Paradigm food is such in its natural, whole-food state, without fortification or addition, or it is not ideal at all.

And so, only if a food has all six characteristics. Only if it is...

* Maximally nutritious

* Innately delicious

* Available and affordable

* Properly prepared

* Environmentally friendly

* Unrefined, unprocessed and whole

...can we call it the perfect food.

FIRST COURSE: MAXIMALLY NUTRITIOUS

For a food to be considered ideal, or Paradigm, it should be maximally nutritious, innately delicious, available and affordable, properly prepared, environmentally friendly, unrefined, unprocessed and whole.

Let us take the characteristics of the ideal food one at a time. First and foremost, food should be maximally nutritious.

Since nutrient content determines nutritional value, let's first look at the nutrients in food.

Calories

Food is made up of calories. A calorie is a unit of energy. So by definition, food is energy.

Practically speaking, a food calorie is the amount of energy a 150-lb person burns each minute while sleeping. There are nearly 1,500 minutes in a day. These calories serve to fuel normal body functions such as breathing and blood flow. In other words, you need to consume, in calories, 10 times your weight in lbs *just to remain alive*. This is called the resting metabolic rate, or RMR.

Unless you are a total couch potato, an additional 500 calories are required for the performance of daily activities, placing the total daily caloric requirement for the average person at 2,000. Conveniently, this corresponds to the amount listed on food labels.

Calorie requirements increase with additional physical activity, as in exercise. For example, running burns approximately 100 calories per mile.[18]

Furthermore, as muscle is more metabolically active than fat, individuals with more lean muscle utilize more calories at rest than those with more fat. It follows that a totally buff dude who runs 10 miles a day could require 3,000 or more calories to satisfy metabolic needs and maintain body weight.

Many people seek out foods or supplements purported to "speed up metabolism" or "burn fat." Maybe you're one of them. If you are, we've got news for you. While it is true that certain vegetables, like cucumbers and celery, are so low in calories that digesting them requires more energy than they supply, not even these "negative calorie foods" can match the impact on metabolism achieved with regular exercise.

Consider that you burn, at rest, **60** calories in one hour. If instead of sitting and watching your favorite sitcom, you were to go outside and run for this same length of time, even at the relatively slow pace of 10 minutes per mile, you would cover six miles and expend **600** calories by the time the show is over. In other words, when you run, your metabolic rate is **10 times** as fast as at rest, and possibly more, as energy expenditure increases progressively at higher speeds. In other *other* words, the faster your run, the more fuel you burn.

Let's look at this another way. In just 3 hours, a running man (or woman) burns the amount of calories (2,000) that it takes a resting person a full 24-hour period to expend. Lesson to be learned: If you want a fast-metabolism, get your move on.

Of course, differences in the genetics, metabolism and behavior of individuals make it difficult to accurately predict a person's caloric requirements. However, you may estimate your caloric needs by multiplying your weight *in kilograms* by **30** if you are sedentary (do not exercise), by **35** if you are moderately active (exercise most days, 30 minutes or less), and by **40** if you are very active (daily exercise, at least 30 minutes per day). One kg equals 2.2 lbs.

Using our 70 kg (154 lb) person as an example, he burns 2,100 calories on days of inactivity, 2,500 calories with moderate activity, and 2,800 calories or more if he exercises vigorously.

As there are 3,500 calories in 1 lb of body weight, and regular vigorous exercise results in a deficit of 700 calories per day, an active individual can expect to burn 1 lb or more of body fat for fuel each week, assuming of course a constant caloric intake.

MACRONUTRIENTS

A calorie's chief purpose is to supply the body with energy. Readily-available, sustained energy.

All things being equal, the extent to which a given calorie fulfills this basic purpose determines its value in the diet.

The three main forms of calories are carbohydrate, protein and fat. They are also called **macronutrients**, and all are present in some amount in most foods.

While all three macronutrients can be used for energy, each fulfills unique functions in your body. What are the functions of the macronutrients?

In general, fat lubricates, insulates, makes hormones and serves as an energy reserve. Dietary fats are made up mainly of fatty-acids.

Protein promotes growth, regenerates tissues and catalyzes chemical reactions. The building blocks for protein are amino acids. There are 20 amino acids available in food, 8 of which are required in the diet. These are the *essential* amino acids.

Carbohydrates consist of simple sugars (glucose and fructose, for example). These occur either on their own, in pairs (lactose, sucrose) or strung together in chains of complex carbohydrates called starch. The simple sugars are distinguished from starch by their sweet taste.

Carbohydrates are the body's primary and preferred source of fuel.

In fact, the brain can use little else but carbohydrates. In order to function properly, your brain requires 140 grams of pure glucose per day, or the amount found in 28 small apples. (A small apple contains 3.5 grams of free glucose and 1.5 gram of glucose in sucrose, for a total of 5 grams of glucose.[19]) If one apple a day keeps the doctor away, 28 may earn you an A. Cheese and meat, on the other hand, have no carbohydrates. Not exactly brain foods, these.

With these and a few other exceptions, most foods contain a mixture of carbohydrate, protein and fat. Exceptions include oil, which is pure fat, table sugar, which is pure carbohydrate, and egg white, which derives all of its calories from protein.

Of the three major macronutrients, fat is the most calorically dense. Fat contains roughly 9 calories per gram, while protein and carbohydrate each contribute about 4 calories per gram. Therefore, a given quantity of fat has over twice as many calories as the same amount of protein or carbohydrate. To illustrate, 1 oz of olive oil (pure fat) contains 250 calories. One oz of pure sugar, which is all carbohydrate, provides 110 calories, or fewer than half the calories present in oil. One oz of watermelon contains under 10 calories. How can watermelon, which like table sugar is mostly carbohydrate, be so low in calories? Because watermelon, by weight, is over 90 percent water, and water is calorie-free. Kind of a food lover's dream. By contrast, sugar and oil, and many animal foods and refined foods, contain little or no water, making them easy to wear around the waist.

Despite the caloric density of fat, carbohydrates predominate as your body's primary source of fuel because the simple sugars present in, for example, fruits and vegetables, are more readily absorbed than the more complex molecules that make up fatty foods, a notion we'll explore in a later section.

A CALORIE IS A CALORIE?

Contrary to the popular belief, all calories are <u>not</u> created equal. Here are some interesting differences.

First, all macronutrients contain atoms of **oxygen, carbon** and **hydrogen**. Protein, however, is the only calorie type that contains **nitrogen**. This is important, because though protein can be used to make carbohydrate and fat, these cannot serve as raw materials for protein, which is required in food. The requirements are small, as we shall see, because your body recycles most proteins from an amino acid pool. Also, unlike the other atoms, nitrogen cannot be stored. Instead, your kidneys must remove excess nitrogen, and this involves a lot of work. The nitrogenous waste appears in your urine mainly in the form of urea, giving the high-protein dieter's pee its characteristic foul smell.

In addition to the burden it places on your kidneys, protein requires the greatest effort of all the macronutrients to convert into fuel. This is known as the **thermic effect of food**. In fact, a high-protein meal requires 3 times as much digestive energy to process as a carbohydrate-rich food and 6 times more energy than fat.[20] This is manifested by an increase in body temperature and is likely due to the greater effort involved in processing the nitrogen in protein, and in converting protein into carbohydrate.

Wait a minute, you may be saying. *I thought food was supposed to give me energy, rather than take my energy away!*

Now you're thinking. While the thermic effect of food results in a temporary increase in your metabolic rate, this energy is wasted as heat rather than being available to, let's say, put a spring in your step, or a smile on your face.

While too much protein can tax the digestive system, too much dietary fat can have the opposite effect. It is not wasted as heat but stored as...you guessed it: fat.

You see, too much of any macronutrient (in excess of caloric needs) is put away for later use in the form of blubber, but none more readily than dietary fat. Storing dietary fat as body fat requires very little energy expenditure (less than 3 calories per 100 calories) and is done within minutes, preferentially around the waist, hips, thighs and buttocks. By contrast, only about 1 percent of ingested carbohydrates end up as body fat.[21]

Okay, up until this point we've talked a lot about energy, calories, and types of calories (protein, fat and carbohydrate). Carbohydrate is your body's preferred energy source and should predominate in the diet, while protein serves to regenerate tissues and fat provides an energy reserve.

But any discussion of energy would be incomplete without a mention of the ultimate energy source. All the energy captured in food derives ultimately from that heavenly orb. You know it. You feel it. You see it (just don't look directly at it). That's right: the sun.

In short, the closer a food is to the sun, the higher the energy yield. Fruits and vegetables receive their energy directly from its glorious rays, none more so than green vegetables. Through chlorophyll and the process of photosynthesis, green vegetables convert the sun's light into carbohydrate, the body's primary energy source. By contrast, animals satisfy their energy requirements by eating plants or in the case of carnivorous fish such as salmon and tuna, other animals. In addition to the carbohydrate in plant food, animals utilize the vitamins and minerals for themselves, and manufacture protein (muscle) and fat. As we will see, with few exceptions, animal products contain few vitamins and minerals and no carbohydrates. In other words, no energy. Instead they are comprised of varying proportions of protein and fat (including cholesterol and saturated fat). Fruits, on the other hand, are packed with pure energy, which is readily available to your body minutes after ingestion. But you probably did not know that fruits also contain protein and fat, as do vegetables. Remember, most foods contain a mix of macronutrients.

What then, you may wonder, is the ideal proportion of carbohydrates, protein and fat in the diet? How much of each do we need? How much should we eat?

Let us take each macronutrient in turn.

FAT

A fat intake comprising roughly 5 percent of total calories efficiently supports physiological processes and assures adequate consumption of the essential fatty acids.

However, because most foods contain more than this amount, and in some cases much more, it is almost impossible to keep dietary fat this low. To prevent disease and maintain a healthy body weight, many physicians recommend a very low fat diet. A very low fat diet derives 10 percent of its calories from fat, which is double the minimum intake of 5 percent.

Some argue that a higher intake of fat (30 percent or more of total calories) may be appropriate for those who wish to gain weight, for athletes and fitness enthusiasts, or for highly active teenagers. If you are in this group, including larger quantities of lipids (fat) in the diet provides concentrated energy for active muscles and does not lead to the weight gain and chronic disease that can occur in sedentary persons on higher-fat diets, especially when high levels of saturated fat are consumed.

Of course, this should not be taken as license to consume copious amounts of oils. Rather, if you are *very lean* and are *very active* or are *actively growing* and find additional dietary fat is required, it should be obtained from whole foods naturally rich in healthy fat, such as avocado and olives. These foods offer the added benefits of fiber, vitamins and minerals, all of which are sorely lacking in oil and butter. *What about nuts?* you ask. Yes, nuts are another high-fat food. While more nutritious than oils, nuts contain lower levels of key nutrients than the vegetable fruits just mentioned, in addition to other drawbacks to be discussed.

Higher fat intakes (in excess of 30 percent of total calories) are associated with high intakes of animal protein, which brings a separate set of health concerns.[22]

The acceptable fat intake, according to the USDA, is between 20 and 35 percent of total calories. The USDA does not set a minimum requirement. The concern is that, because fat is so calorically-dense, reducing intake may cause a negative energy balance and result in unintentional weight loss. In other words, if you simply cut fat out of the diet without replacing it with other macronutrients, your caloric intake may fall to levels insufficient to meet your energy needs. This at least is the concern. While this may be theoretically true, in practice it never happens. Take for example the Chinese, whose dietary fat intake is low (under 15 percent) and whose energy needs are easily met with carbohydrates found plentifully in fruits, vegetables and beans. Moreover, the risk of cancer goes *up* with higher intakes of dietary fat, starting at levels of 40 grams per day, which is roughly 20 percent of calories on a 2,000-calorie diet.[23]

In summary, a diet consisting of 5 percent fat meets our minimum needs, 10 percent is recommended to reverse and prevent disease, and your risk for cancer starts increasing on diets of 20 percent fat. In fact, doubling fat intake from 20 percent to 40 percent is associated with a 15 percent increased risk of breast cancer.[24] Therefore the USDA's *minimum* recommendation (20 percent) should actually be the *maximum* fat content advisable, if of course your goal is to enjoy good health. This is never more true than if you consume animal products, which have an additive effect on your risk for chronic conditions, and also tend to derive a large portion of their calories from fat.

So if a diet of 10 percent fat prevents disease, and a diet of over 20 percent increases your risk of health problems, how much fat am I taking in each day? you ask. The average fat intake in the standard American diet is about 40 percent. No wonder everyone's so sick!

It is a fact not widely understood that the fat naturally occurring in fruits and vegetables is more than adequate to meet the needs of most everyone.

Even those foods commonly considered fat-free, such as broccoli, lemons and bell peppers, derive 10 percent of their calories from fat. In fact, it is hard to find a vegetable that is not at least 10 percent fat. Spinach and Romaine lettuce are approximately 15 percent fat. Olives and avocados? Seventy-five percent fat.

You do not need to be a math whiz to understand that if you spend your days eating vegetables, most of which are 10 percent fat, your overall fat intake is...you guessed it: 10 percent. Your needs have easily been met, without a spot of butter, a drop of oil, a bag of nuts or a breast of chicken. With fat ever-present in foods, the concern should not be on getting enough in your diet, but on avoiding too much. As a source of concentrated calories and deficient in nutrients relative to foods rich in carbohydrates, high-fat foods are too easily overeaten, and when they are, the excess is quickly and efficiently turned into...you got it: fat.

Types of Fat

Let's spend a moment discussing the types of fat present in food.

Dietary fats include triglycerides, cholesterol and free fatty acids. Triglycerides are far and away the most abundant breed of fat in foods. As the name suggests, triglycerides contain three (tri) fatty acids attached to a molecule of glycerol, which is a type of alcohol. Triglycerides are classified based on their constituent fatty acids, which can be saturated, unsaturated and trans fats. Fatty acids are distinguished by the presence and number of double bonds they contain. Saturated fats contain no double bonds, while unsaturated fats contain one (mono) or more than one (poly) double bond. This has to do with how many carbon and hydrogen atoms are present, which in turn determines the temperature at which a fat melts. But really, memorizing the chemical nature of various fats matters less than identifying the type of fat your diet should feature. After all, we're not going to quiz you. You get an A just for reading.

As we shall see, the healthiest diet emphasizes certain unsaturated fats while minimizing cholesterol, saturated fat and trans fat.

First, the unsaturated fats.

Unsaturated fats include monounsaturated (*mono*) and polyunsaturated (*poly*) varieties. These fats occur together in varying proportions in most foods. Foods such as olives and avocados have more mono than poly. Most fruits and vegetables, including lemons, broccoli, spinach and apples, have more poly than mono.

Next, the polyunsaturated fats.

Polyunsaturated fats include omega-3 (n-3) and omega-6 (n-6) fatty acids. These are essential fats. As with vitamins and minerals, your body cannot produce them, so you must consume them in food.

These two types of polyunsaturated fats have opposing effects. In general, omega-6s increase inflammation and pain, while omega-3s have natural anti-inflammatory effects and protect the heart. Moreover, omega-3s are concentrated in the brain and modulate mood, memory and attention.

What is inflammation? Robbins *Pathologic Basis of Disease* tells us it is the body's reaction to invaders. These invaders can be bacteria, toxins or foreign particles such as dirt and splinters, which are not supposed to be in you and can potentially harm you.[25]

Inflammation is characterized by *tumor* (swelling), *dolor* (pain), *rubor* (redness), *calor* (warmth) and *functio laesa* (loss of function) and occurs when you get cut, scraped or fall and hit your head. The swelling, warmth and redness are your body's way of protecting itself, by getting rid of both the initial cause of injury (infection or chemical exposure) and the consequences of such injury (dead cells and tissues). The pain tells you to leave the area alone while it heals. The loss of function is an inconvenient consequence of the swelling and pain, but serves a protective function by allowing wounds to heal.

While its fundamental goal is protective, the inflammatory response can in some instances actually do more harm than good.

Imagine your body as a battlefield. The forces of evil are toxins and microbes. The forces of good are the cells of your immune system. When bacteria invade, your immune cells attack, guns ablaze and hand grenades booming. The two opposing forces do battle and casualties arise on both sides. Dead bodies litter the ground. Amidst all the explosion and blood and guts, damage to the surrounding houses, buildings and parks is an inevitable consequence. These structures are your blood vessels, skin and joints. The battlefield is you. And if your own infantry is too heavily armed or mounts too aggressive a response, they end up harming the very territory they are employed to protect.

This is not to say that inflammation is not necessary and good. Without it, that pesky cough would never go away, that razor nick would never heal and that newly pierced ear would remain a permanently festering sore. Luckily, the inflammatory response is closely connected with the process of repair. Inflammation's infantry walls off and destroys the invaders, and in the process of repair, scar tissue replaces injured tissue. It is only when inflammatory reactions go unchecked that problems arise. This underlies common conditions such as arthritis and atherosclerosis (fatty plaques), as well as excessive reactions to insect bites, drugs and toxins. These *inflammatory* conditions are increasingly more common. If you or a friend has ever swollen up after eating a particular food or getting stung by a bee, you have seen or experienced an unchecked inflammatory response for yourself.

What causes excessive inflammation? Diet is a big contributor. Omega-6, present in so many dietary staples, feeds the inflammatory response, causing it to run in the red. Your body turns omega-6 into a chemical called arachidonic acid (AA), which gives rise to prostaglandins (PGs).

Gosh, all these multi-syllables!

PGs and related compounds mediate every step of inflammation and are especially involved in the pain response. Excessive PGs can result in pain that is out of proportion to the level of tissue damage. This can occur, for example, in chronic pain conditions such as fibromyalgia in which there is no evidence of injury but whose sufferers nevertheless experience severe, incapacitating pain.

As the standard American diet has relied more and more heavily on plant oils, grains, grain-fed meat and nuts, the inflammatory response has spun out of control in more and more people. For this reason anti-inflammatory drugs such as aspirin and Advil are so popular: They suppress your body's already revved-up immune response and bring it back to normal, so that a less aggressive attack is waged, less damage is done, and less scar tissue is formed. But these medications have harmful side effects, not the least of which include stomach ulcers, gastrointestinal bleeding and kidney damage, as well as difficulty breathing and worsening of asthma. It would be nice if a natural source of anti-inflammatory existed, say, in food.

Enter omega-3s. Your body is unable to convert omega-3 fatty acids into PGs at the same rate that it can generate these pain-makers from omega-6s. Consequently, less inflammation occurs and less pain is experienced. A natural pain-reliever, present in food. Well, in certain foods.

Before the rise of processed foods, humans ate equal amounts of each type of essential fatty acid. In other words, the ratio of omega-6 to omega-3 in the diet was roughly 1:1.[26]

However, because omega-6 is present in greater abundance in most modern foods, it is nearly impossible to consume as much omega-3 as omega-6, and the current recommendations reflect this. In fact, the USDA recommends a ratio of omega-6 to 3 that is 10 to 1. In the average diet, with its reliance on oils, grains, grain-fed meat and nuts, the ratio actually consumed is closer to 20 to 1 and may be higher. Consider that 1 cup of oatmeal contains 1,800 mg of omega-6 and only 80 mg of omega-3, a ratio of over 20 to 1. One serving (2 tbsp) of peanut butter has 4,500 mg of omega-6 and only 25 mg of omega-3, a ratio of 180 to 1 favoring omega-6, and disfavoring health.

The imbalance between omega-3 and omega-6 fatty acids may explain the rise of such diseases as asthma, autoimmune conditions such as arthritis, lupus and multiple sclerosis, as well as heart disease, cancer, Type 2 diabetes and Alzheimer's, all of which are inflammatory. Too much omega-6 and not enough omega-3 may also contribute to obesity, depression, dyslexia, hyperactivity and even a tendency toward violence.[27] Lay on your horn much?

If it is a good idea to eat more omega-3, in which foods are they found? Omega-3 fatty acids come in three varieties.

ALA (Alpha-Linolenic Acid) is found in plant foods (leafy greens and seeds).

EPA (Eicosopentaenoic Acid) and **DHA** (Docosahexaenoic Acid) are derived from ALA and found in animals, mainly in fatty fish.

In healthy individuals who exclude animal products from their diet, the body is able to convert ALA to EPA and DHA, which makes ALA the only true essential omega-3. Individuals who are insulin resistant, overweight or have high blood pressure or high cholesterol, or eat large amounts of omega-6 fats, may find it necessary to obtain EPA and DHA from the diet. For these folks, and for those who happen to like the taste, seaweed is a worthy source.

The recommended dietary intake of roughly 1,000 mg of omega-3 is to offset the huge amount of omega-6 in the average diet. **It is wise to reduce or eliminate foods such as nuts, oils, grains and meat, all of which have disproportionately large amounts of omega-6, in favor of foods with healthier ratios.**

Which foods might these be?

In many fruits and vegetables, the ratio is actually reversed. One head of Romaine lettuce, for instance, contains over twice as much omega-3 as omega-6 (700 mg to 300 mg). Three cups of boiled spinach contains 5 times more omega-3 than 6 (800 mg to 150 mg). Taken together, 3 cups of boiled spinach and 1 head of Romaine lettuce provide 1.5 grams of omega-3s, which fulfills the daily requirement, *at a mere 300 calories.*

There are other sources of omega-3. One oz of walnuts, for example, contains 2,500 mg. However, walnuts have over four times more omega-6. Fatty fish such as salmon is also high in omega-3, but as we shall see fish contains a variety of other ingredients, including saturated fat, cholesterol, pollutants and toxic metals. These are, shall we say, less than Paradigm.

Some argue that even in healthy individuals, the body may only convert 10 percent of dietary ALA to EPA and DHA, and so in vegetarians, vegans and others who abstain from fish, higher quantities of ALA may be necessary. However, because the same enzyme used to turn ALA into EPA and DHA (desaturase, for your info) also converts omega-6s to inflammatory prostaglandins, reducing the amount of omega-6s in the diet frees up the enzyme to get to work making EPA and DHA and makes it unlikely that plant-eaters need to add huge amounts of ALA (measured in grams).

That being said, if you wish to include more omega-3 in your diet, a wise choice would be to consume flax or chia seeds. Two tbsp of ground flax contains 3,000 mg of omega-3 and just 800 mg of omega-6. These seeds are savory and go well blended into smoothies and sprinkled over salads.

To summarize, polyunsaturated fats come in two classes. Omega-6s are found in nuts, animal products, grains and vegetable oils. They are essential in small doses but if consumed in excessive amounts are pro-inflammatory, disease-producing and pain-causing. Omega-3 is found in leafy green vegetables, seeds and seaweed. It promotes health but is generally consumed in insufficient amounts. It is wise therefore to include large quantities of dark, leafy green vegetables and perhaps 1 or 2 tbsp of chia and/or flax seeds in your daily diet, along with monounsaturated fats found for example in olives and avocados.

The other types of fats - saturated fats, trans fats and cholesterol - are NOT required in the diet and can be harmful if not deadly.

Cholesterol

Contrary to what you may have heard, cholesterol is not all bad. Yes, high concentrations in your blood can clog your arteries and damage your heart and brain. But cholesterol serves several important functions. It helps to keep your cell membranes together. It regulates the passage of molecules into your cells. It helps you absorb dietary fat. Cholesterol is also used to create sex hormones including testosterone and estrogen, as well as vitamin D. The problem is not with cholesterol per se, but with how much you consume, and most people, in fact everyone except those who shun all animal products including eggs and dairy, eat too much.

This is because your liver manufactures enough cholesterol to satisfy all physiological processes and so obtaining any in the diet is unnecessary and can contribute to fatty plaques (remember those?) and weight gain. Cholesterol is derived exclusively from animal products – meat, fish, eggs and dairy. Plant foods – fruits, vegetables, beans and seeds – are naturally cholesterol-free.

Saturated Fat

Your body uses saturated fats for structural purposes, and your nervous system (brain, spinal cord) contains an abundance. As with cholesterol, your body is able synthesize saturated fat and so it is not essential to obtain it in food.

Dietary saturated fat is solid at room temperature. It is found in meat, dairy and fried foods (often in the form of pig fat, or lard), as well as in vegetable oils. Saturated fat is present in negligible amounts in most fruits and vegetables. Exceptions are chocolate and coconut, which are high in saturated fat. A dark chocolate bar contains over 8 grams; a tbsp of coconut oil has nearly 12 grams.

The USDA recommends keeping saturated fat intake as low as you can. Because it is present in so many foods, eliminating it from the diet entirely is impossible. The upper limit for recommended saturated fat is 20 grams per day in the average diet, i.e. one consisting of 2,000 calories and 30 percent fat. In a diet of 10 percent fat, this value is about 7 grams daily, or the amount of saturated fat present in 2 avocados, 4 cups of olives, 4 tbsp of peanut butter, 4 oz of steak, 2 slices of cheese, or ½ tbsp of coconut oil. Note how saturated fat is concentrated in animal products. High intakes of saturated fat are associated with weight gain, heart disease, high blood pressure and cerebral vascular disease (stroke). As none of these conditions is desirable, saturated fat should be shunned.

If you require more incentive to say NO to saturated fat, consider that both saturated fat and cholesterol trigger the arachidonic acid cascade (AA, remember?) and increase the degree of inflammation in your body.[28] These mini explosions damage joints, blood vessels and are at the root of autoimmune diseases.

Since cholesterol and saturated fat often exist in the same foods (animal foods), and in high amounts in these foods, they can be said to team up to hijack health.

Therefore, efforts should be made to limit cholesterol and saturated fat consumption, with a goal of zero cholesterol and under 10 grams of saturated fat per day.

How to achieve this with ease? Easy as 1, 2, 3, as we shall see.

Trans fats

Trans fats (partially-hydrogenated vegetable oils) are a chemically-altered, man-made entity synthesized in the laboratory by adding hydrogen to vegetable oils (omega-6 fats) and exposing them to high heat. This makes them solid at room temperature and prolongs their shelf life. A manufacturer's dream is a physiological nightmare.

Trans fats do not exist in nature and they do not exist in you, not naturally at least. In contrast to cholesterol and saturated fat, trans fats serve no beneficial purpose in your body. Your system suffers to recognize and dispose of them. These fats can be found in margarine, many brands of peanut butter, baked goods, deep-fried foods and some salad dressings. Trans fats clog the blood and ruin the body and the brain. They contribute to Alzheimer's dementia.[29] In addition, those whose diets include trans fats experience increased weight gain and abdominal fat compared to those with similar caloric intakes and no trans fats. Derived from omega-6 fatty acids, trans fats promote pain and inflammation, which can lead to chronic disease and make life a real bummer.

To reiterate, there is absolutely no benefit to trans fats, which are poisonous. Any intake, even one seemingly harmless bite of a doughnut, is by definition too much. If your wish is to kill yourself, better to drink strychnine. It is quick and painless, which cannot be said for the heart disease, cancer and stroke that inevitably ensue from the consumption of trans fat foods. If your body is able to rid these fats from your blood before they explode in your arteries, it simply stores them as belly flab.[30] That's a real bummer.

Together, trans fats, cholesterol and saturated fatty acids, and excessive amounts of omega-6 fatty acids, deserve to be called **nasty fats**.

In order to maximize health, emphasize monounsaturated fats and omega-3 fats found in sweets, greens, beans and seeds.

FAT CHEAT SHEET

Omega-3 fats: good for you; found in leafy greens, seaweed, seeds (flax/chia)

Monounsaturated fats: good for you; found in olives and avocados

Omega-6 fats: required in small amounts but consumed excessively in most diets; found in vegetables oils, grains, nuts and animal products

Cholesterol: unnecessary in the diet; found in animal foods

Saturated fat: unnecessary in the diet; found in animal foods, chocolate and certain vegetable oils (coconut, palm kernel)

Trans fat: deadly; found in margarine, baked goods, fried-foods, partially-hydrogenated oils

PROTEIN

As for protein, not all authorities agree on a precise figure for our daily needs. The calculations of impartial experts fall within a range that runs from as little as 2 ½ percent[31] to as much as 10 percent.

At the higher end of this range is the USDA, which recommends a daily protein intake of 56 grams for men and 46 grams for women, which is just under 10 percent of calories on a 2,000 to 2,500-calorie diet. If you are between the ages of 9 and 13, the recommendation is 34 grams of protein per day. To complicate matters further, the USDA adds to its recommendation an acceptable range of protein intake, which is between 10 and 35 percent of total calories (likely to allow if not encourage the consumption of government-subsidized foods including beef, eggs and dairy, which are high in protein).

So, who is right?

Since no consensus exists, not even within the same regulatory agency, let us use common sense.

Mother's milk, arguably nature's perfect food at a time when we, as infants, grow more rapidly than any other period of life, contains only 5 percent protein.

That is correct: 5 percent.

There is simply no physiological advantage to making protein more than 5 or at most 10 percent of the diet, which is 50 grams per 2,000 calories. In fact, there may be deadly disadvantages. Animal protein, whether consumed as meat or milk, acidifies the blood, weakens the bones and damages the kidneys. Animal protein also promotes the development of cancer, more so if consumed in excess of 10 percent of total calories, as recent studies such as those undertaken by researchers at Cornell University have shown.[32]

The food pyramid, developed by the Department of Agriculture and available at MyPyramid.gov, recommends that adult men consume 6 oz of meat and 3 cups of milk. This alone contributes over 15 percent of calories to a 2,000 calorie diet. Clearly, the USDA has not caught up with the latest research. Nor have most Americans, who consume an average of 15 to 16 percent of calories from protein, mostly in the form of animal foods.

Plant protein, even in amounts as high as 20 percent of total calories - which corresponds to the amount found in many legumes (kidney beans, for example) - does not pose these health risks.

Protein Quality

Clearly, all protein is not created equal. Animal protein poses health risks, while plant protein promotes health.

But I thought animal protein was a complete protein. Complete is better, right?

Oh, yes, what about complete protein?

In order for a protein to be called *complete*, it must contain all essential amino acids. These amino acids your body does not produce and are therefore required in the diet. Complete proteins contain them in their proper proportions. In other words, in the proportions similar to what occurs in the human body. (The most complete protein is human flesh, but eating one's neighbor is considered taboo and not recommended.)

A common misconception is that the only complete protein is meat. It is true that many animal foods, including eggs and milk, are complete proteins. However, all foods that contain protein have at least some amount of all essential amino acids, and many plant foods contain them in their proper proportions. Soybeans, for instance, are complete proteins. Many green vegetables, including spinach and broccoli, are also high in all essential amino acids. In fact, gorillas, whose anatomy and physiology closely resemble our own, and whose genetic code (DNA) is virtually identical, derive the bulk of their protein from green vegetation. No one can doubt the size and strength of our furry-chested friends. And green vegetables, like many beans, derive a large portion of their calories from protein. For example, spinach is 49 percent protein; Brussels sprouts, broccoli and kale each contain about 45 percent protein.[33]

Cauliflower, which is not commonly considered a high-protein food, is 40 percent protein. By comparison, a whole egg is only 35 percent protein. Low-fat milk, only 26 percent.

Wait a minute, we hear you saying. *You mean to tell me that cauliflower has more protein than milk?* Yes, and more than eggs too.

Cauliflower and other vegetables are also much higher than animal foods in almost all nutrients, including the minerals iron and calcium. For example, 100 calories (1.5 oz) of steak contains a mere 4 percent of the daily value (DV) of iron and only 1 percent of the DV of calcium. Ten oz of milk (100 calories) has 1 percent of the DV of iron and 38 percent of the DV for calcium.

By comparison, 100 calories of spinach meets 90 percent of the average person's iron requirement and 60 percent of the daily value of calcium.

Wait, spinach has more calcium than milk and more iron than red meat? Yes.

Not only does spinach have more calcium than milk and more iron than red meat, the iron in spinach is in a healthier form. Heme iron, which is present in meat, acts as an oxidant. Oxidants are free radicals. This type of iron hastens cell death and aging if consumed in excess of your body's requirement. By contrast, the non-heme iron found in plants is only assimilated in the amounts required by your body. The remainder is excreted by your kidneys. Though less efficiently absorbed than its heme counterpart, non-heme iron is helped into the bloodstream by vitamin C, an antioxidant found in abundance in plant foods. Animal products do not contain vitamin C.

Although the terms *complete* and *high-quality* are sometimes used interchangeably when applied to protein, they should not be thought of as synonymous. As we have discussed, *complete* refers to the amino acid sequence of a particular protein. *High-quality*, on the other hand, refers to a protein's growth-promoting capability. While both soybeans and eggs are complete proteins, eggs and other animal foods are more growth-promoting than plant foods, in that they cause cells to divide more rapidly. But it is not just muscles that they build. Animal foods stimulate the production of growth hormones, including Insulin-like Growth Factor 1 (IGF-1), which contribute to cancer and obesity.[343536]

It follows, then, that if the growth of one's waist size not to mention many deadly tumors is what is meant by the term "high quality," we would do well, in the case of protein, to confine ourselves to plants.

Even for those such as bodybuilders and professional athletes who may require additional protein to replace exercise-induced losses and build muscle, the body can derive all the essential amino acids from the natural variety of plant proteins that we encounter every day.

It was once believed that you needed to combine incomplete proteins in such a way as to overcome deficiencies and supply adequate amounts of all essential amino acids. Frances Moore Lappe popularized this notion in her book, *Diet for a Small Planet.* This is simply not the case, and Ms. Lappe retracted this assertion in a later edition of the book, but the myth has lived on.

Let's bury it once and for all.

Protein complementarity is irrelevant. Even foods deemed incomplete or deficient in one amino acid or another can, if eaten in sufficient amounts, supply your body's protein requirement completely. Case in point: Kidney beans are said to be incomplete because they are a poor source of the essential amino acid methionine. For this reason, it is advisable to combine beans with wheat, which is methionine rich, in order to "produce a complete protein of improved biologic value."[37] But let us analyze this statement. The essential amino acids are histidine, isoleucine, leucine, lysine, methionine (and cysteine, in some), phenylalanine (and possibly tyrosine), threonine, tryptophan and valine.

According to the World Health Organization, the daily requirements for these amino acids, for a 70 kg (154 lb) person are as follows.[38]

histidine:	700 mg
isoleucine:	1,400 mg
leucine:	2,800 mg
lysine:	2,100 mg
methionine:	700 mg
cysteine:	350 mg
phenylalanine + tyrosine:	1,750 mg
threonine:	1,050 mg
tryptophan:	280 mg
valine:	1,820 mg

Do you really need to combine proteins, or eat complete proteins at every meal or every day to achieve this intake of the essential amino acids? Hmmm, let us test this notion by choosing kidney beans, a so-called *incomplete* protein, and imagining a day in which we eat nothing but kidney beans. A bit monotonous, yes, but if such an intake yields the daily requirement of all essential amino acids, we have disproved the protein complementarity myth and shown that food combining is hogwash.

Eating 2,000 calories worth of kidney beans, equivalent to 9.5 cups cooked, provides the following quantities of essential amino acids:[39]

histidine:	3,500 mg
isoleucine:	6,000 mg
leucine:	10,800 mg
lysine:	8,925 mg
methionine:	1,650 mg
cysteine:	1,200 mg
phenylalanine + tyrosine:	10,500 mg
threonine:	4,700 mg
tryptophan:	1,500 mg
valine:	7,350 mg

As you can see, though considered incomplete, kidney beans provide huge amounts of all 10 essential amino acids, in some cases over 5 times the minimum recommended intake. Are they deficient in methionine, as the textbooks say? Actually, no. Kidney beans provide over twice the daily requirement for methionine. Take that to your next meal.

We won't belabor the point, but you are welcome to try this experiment yourself. Choose potatoes, which like beans are considered incomplete, and see for yourself whether eating nothing but potatoes satisfies your protein requirements. (Hint: It does.)

In summary, plant protein, even those sources deemed incomplete, provides all essential amino acids in quantities great enough to fulfill your body's needs. There is no need to choose certain combinations or to supplement with animal foods. There is also no value to your body in consuming more than 10 percent of your calories from protein. Excessive amounts are simply made into *waste* or worn around your *waist*. Hopefully the USDA will catch on and tailor the recommendations accordingly. Unfortunately, whether by choice or by convention, too many Americans are following the advice of this government agency, judging by the prevalence of osteoporosis, kidney stones, high blood pressure and cancer, all of which are diseases of protein excess.

CARBOHYDRATES

If, then, the ideal diet is low in fat (10 percent) and low in protein (10 percent), the remainder, or roughly 80 percent of total calories, derives from carbohydrates. As with protein and fats, not all carbohydrates are created equal. The ideal carbohydrate comes packaged in **water** and **fiber**, which slows its absorption, stabilizes blood sugar levels and provides sustained energy.

Let's look at the different carbohydrates by first identifying what they have in common.

All carbohydrates are comprised of the simple sugars, fructose and glucose. (Galactose, which is found in milk, is the third type of simple sugar.) These sugars can exist freely in foods, attached in pairs, or strung together in long chains. For example, the disaccharide sucrose, otherwise known as table sugar, is composed of equal parts fructose and glucose. Lactose, or milk sugar, is made up of glucose and galactose. Of note, in early childhood, many of us lose the ability to digest milk sugar. In some Black and Asian populations, the rate of lactose intolerance, as this is called, is as high as 90 percent.

Long chains of glucose molecules are called complex carbohydrates, also known as starch. They are found in foods such as beans, grains, nuts, peas and potatoes.

Whether free, in pairs, or in longer chains, fructose and glucose are part of virtually every carbohydrate food. Even fruits, which are a major source of fructose in the diet, contain an equal amount of glucose. And many vegetables including spinach and broccoli contain glucose.

Though fructose and glucose are both simple sugars and appear in many of the same foods, they are actually handled quite differently by the digestion. To begin with, the rate of fructose metabolism is more rapid than that of glucose. And unlike glucose, fructose does not stimulate the secretion of insulin, a hormone involved in weight gain, water retention and fat storage. Of course, sucking down loads of pure fructose, whether in fruit juice or in soft drinks, can lead to health problems. A mix of fructose and glucose, packaged with water and fiber as occurs in fruits and vegetables, provides sustained energy with little digestive effort and is therefore a preferred form of dietary carbohydrate.

And so, in a 2,000-calorie diet, 80 percent of calories should derive from carbohydrate (1,600 calories, 400 grams); 10

percent of calories from protein (200 calories, 50 grams); and 10 percent of calories from fat (200 calories, roughly 25 grams).

These ratios correspond nicely to the eating patterns of the world's longest lived peoples, those of Russia, Ecuador and Pakistan who boast life spans that routinely break the century mark. The elders of these peoples remain healthy, active, alert and vigorous well into old age. Their diets contain, on average, roughly 10 percent protein, 15 percent fat and the remainder carbohydrates.[40]

If these percentages and quantities are hard to remember, and you prefer not to spend your days with calculator in hand determining the nutrient breakdown of everything that enters your mouth, you are not alone. We are the same, and so is the bulk of the human race. You'll be happy to know that some foods naturally contain the correct macronutrient ratios, and by emphasizing these foods at every meal, you insure that your overall intake is in line with these proportions. For as they say, as the part, so the whole.

But first, let's analyze these figures.

How much is 25 grams of fat? A lot, if the source is fruits or vegetables. Spinach is 14 percent fat, and yet you'd have to eat over 1,500 calories of boiled spinach (40 cups) to approach 25 grams of fat. In contrast, if you eat animal protein or other concentrated foods, 25 grams of fat is yours in only a few small bites. This much fat is found in 5 eggs, 2 ½ slices of cheese pizza, or 1 Big Mac. Two oz of almonds, or two tbsp of olive oil, each has 25 grams of fat. Spinach comes packaged in water and fiber; animal foods are loaded with saturated fat and cholesterol.

As for protein, it is well-nigh impossible *not* to get enough. Almost any food can meet the daily requirement of 50 grams. We have already mentioned several excellent sources of plant protein, but there are many others that often go unrecognized. Lettuce, for example, derives 34 percent of its calories from protein. Cucumbers are 24 percent protein. Potatoes have 11 percent protein. Fruits are not commonly noted for their protein power; however if you were to eat nothing but lemons all day, you'd achieve 15 percent of your total calories from protein (over 30 grams on a 2,000 calorie diet). A diet exclusively of melons such as honeydew and cantaloupe would also meet your protein requirement.

Too much protein, on the other hand, is far too easily obtainable in the standard American diet (SAD). S-A-D sad. It is sad! Fifty grams of protein is easy to exceed if you eat animal products.

For example, one can of tuna has over 40 grams of protein. One medium chicken breast has nearly 60 grams. You could skip breakfast and have a chicken breast sandwich for lunch and you'd be in the protein red before your evening meal. And it gets more outrageous still: One salmon filet has nearly 80 grams of protein. What happens to the excess protein? As mentioned, it weakens the bones, contributes to the formation of kidney stones, encourages tumor growth and causes weight gain.

PARADIGM PROPORTIONS

What foods in nature approximate this ideal ratio of 80 percent carbohydrates to 10 percent protein to 10 percent fat (80-10-10)?

As mentioned, animal products do not contain any carbohydrates. Hence, they are a very poor source of energy. Meat, eggs and dairy contain varying ratios of protein to fat. For example, canned tuna is 95 percent protein and 5 percent fat (0-95-5). Chicken breast is 65 percent protein, 35 percent fat (0-65-35). Butter contains no protein or carbohydrate. It is pure fat (0-0-100).

Like butter, all oils are 100 percent fat (0-0-100).

Nuts and seeds have little carbohydrate. Rather, they contain a ratio that is skewed in favor of fat, the remainder equally divided between protein and carbohydrate. Almonds are roughly 15-15-70.

All grains are mainly (70 to 90 percent) carbohydrate. Oats, for example, are 70-15-15.

Like grains, legumes (beans, peas, lentils) are mostly carbohydrate, but with a higher percentage of protein. Lentils contain a ratio of roughly 70-25-5.

With few exceptions, fruits are practically pure energy, as they contain about 90 percent carbohydrate, 5 percent protein, and 5 percent fat (90-5-5). Olives and avocados have more fat.

Vegetables have more protein than fruit, green vegetables especially. We've mentioned many of them. Green beans, for example, have 13 percent protein. Red pepper, a vegetable fruit and perhaps nature's perfect food, is exactly 80-10-10.

From this, it would seem that a diet containing a mixture of fruit and vegetables best approximates and in some cases achieves exactly the proper proportion of macronutrients. Some fruits may be a little low in protein and fat, but including beans and seeds increases your intake of these macronutrients and puts your diet in the Paradigm range.

WATER AND FIBER

Though calorie-free, these two essential nutrients are big-time players and should not be ignored. Acting synergistically, water and fiber promote gastrointestinal health. If either is absent from a food, that food is more difficult to digest, its nutrients inefficiently absorbed, and regardless of how many vitamins and minerals it may have, it is therefore deficient. (This, we'll see, is the case with nuts.)

Fiber is defined as the nondigestible portion of plants. Because the human body lacks the enzymes to break it down, fiber generally remains in the gastrointestinal tract and never makes its way into your bloodstream. However, bacteria in your intestinal tract are able to ferment fiber and resistant starch into short-chain fatty acids (SCFAs). SCFAs are the **preferred energy source** for colonocytes (cells of your colon). These highly metabolically active cells are responsible for moving food through your tract. Without the fuel derived from fiber, colonocytes are unable to properly perform their function, become leaky, and toxins that would otherwise be excreted in feces are absorbed into your blood, which is, er, not so good. Additionally, SCFAs help lower inflammation in your intestinal tract and they have anti-tumor effects, protecting against colon cancer.[41]

Because of its numerous health benefits, the National Academy of Sciences lumps fiber into the same group as the other macronutrients, even though it is calorie-free.[42]

What's so beneficial about fiber? Glad you asked. Fiber stabilizes blood sugar and keeps your energy levels steady; it supports intestinal motility by adding bulk to the stool. In addition, fiber lowers cholesterol and reduces your risk of constipation, hemorrhoids and certain forms of cancer.

If you think these benefits are for fogies, you may be interested in this: Fiber makes you feel fuller faster and for longer periods, so that you can eat more food, take in fewer calories, and remain lean - but hopefully not mean. Also, because high fiber diets are associated with less straining on the potty, you can kiss your risk of varicose veins goodbye. None of those blue spider webs for you!

As with the simple sugars, fiber comes in two varieties, and they tend to occur in the same foods. *Insoluble* fiber does not dissolve in water. Instead, it passes through your digestive tract intact, acting like a rake to move debris through you. *Soluble* fiber combines with water to form a viscous gel in your gut. In fact, it is able to absorb 10 times its weight in water. Let's inspect this statement. A large apple contains 5 grams of fiber. Once it reaches your small intestine, this fiber can combine with water, either in the fruit itself or from the glass you had with lunch, to multiply its weight by 10. Suddenly 5 grams has become 50 grams. This added bulk in your gut may keep you from grabbing for that 50-gram doughnut, which saves you from the 200 empty calories and 10 grams of fat that this sweet nothing provides. Let's hear it for fiber! Unfortunately, most people haven't gotten the message.

It is recommended to get at least 25 grams of fiber a day. The average daily intake of fiber in the United States? A paltry 10 grams.

Incidentally, there is no limit to how much fiber you can consume, other than the ability of your intestinal tract to expand without exploding. Fiber's benefits are seen in diets containing 100 grams a day or more. Additionally, fiber and fat show an inverse relationship. As your intake of one goes up, your intake of the other goes down. This is because foods high in fat are generally low in fiber (animal foods), while foods high in fiber tend to be low in fat (fruits, vegetables, beans).

Fiber content varies by food group. By far, fruits, vegetables and legumes have the highest fiber contents of all foods. **Per 100 calories, lentils have 7 grams of fiber, spinach has 10 grams and raspberries contain 12.5 grams.** The other food groups make modest if any contributions to your fiber intake. Per 100 calories, oats have 2.5 grams. Walnuts have about 1 gram. Animal products and oils have no fiber.

Considering fiber's lack of calories and abundance of health benefits, assuring an adequate intake should be atop your to-do list. Stop being preoccupied with protein and focus on fiber. Your gastrointestinal tract, whose health determines the health of your entire body, depends on it.

Clearly, the easiest way to increase fiber consumption is by eating more fruits and vegetables.

What about bran? you may ask. *And high-fiber bread?*

The problems with these foods are several. Often, the source of the fiber is psyllium husk or oat bran, which are hardly edible. Indeed, they look and taste like cardboard. Better to save your money and munch on a UPS box. Also, these fiber types lack the vitamins and minerals present in whole fruits or vegetables. Instead of buying

Metamucil, with its paltry 3 grams of fiber per serving, treat yourself to a box of raspberries (12.5 grams of fiber), or grab an apple or two (8 grams of fiber).

A final problem with processed fibers is their lack of water content. Ever had a dry mouth after eating a piece of bread or cereal bar? Here's why: Fiber requires water to properly move food through the gut. If there is no water present in the food itself, it borrows it from your bloodstream. To replace the water lost from your blood, your cells donate some of theirs, causing them to shrivel and lose their function (we're being extreme, but still). This goes for dried fruit as well, which contains a very small amount of water compared with the fresh version. Take raisins versus grapes, for instance. One cup of raisins, at 434 calories, contains 22 grams of water, just under one oz. Fresh grapes, on the other hand, contain 5.5 times as much water, at only one-fourth of the calories. Per calorie, fresh grapes have over 20 times as much water as shriveled up raisins. Eating 434 calories of grapes is equivalent to drinking 2 large glasses of water (18 oz), which you don't get with raisins. While dried fruit is an excellent source of fiber and certainly preferable to bran, oats, psyllium and other pack-aged processed sources, choose fresh fruit first, and if it's dry fruit you crave, consume it with juicy fruits, or drink it down with water.

Speaking of water, this most precious resource on Earth is the essence of life. It happens to serve a few physiological functions as well. Water catalyzes chemical reactions, transports nutrients, bathes your cells and lubricates your joints. It regulates temperature, moisturizes your skin, supports proper bowel function, cleanses and detoxifies. You can last several weeks without food, but only a few days without water.

How much of your diet should be made up of water? The human body consists of nearly 70 percent water, even more in thin individuals. It follows by analogy that 70 percent of the dietary in-take, by weight, be in the form of water.

To replace the amount lost through urination, perspiration, breathing and bowel movements, authorities recommend 8 to 12 eight-oz glasses of water (64 to 96 total oz, or 2 to 3 L), and possibly more depending on the weather and one's activity level.[43] This rec-ommendation is based on the standard American diet (so SAD), which is high in animal foods and refined grains, both of which con-tain very little water.

(To test the validity of this, conduct an experiment of your own: Put a chicken breast, or a bagel, through a juicer and note the absence of any liquid whatsoever. Compare this with one large apple, which is 85 percent water and yields nearly a cup of juice. *Better yet, don't try this and just trust us.*)

Since the typical foods are so dry, the estimation is that only 20 percent of our water comes from the food we eat, and therefore 80 percent should come from beverages. But when consumed with meals, water dilutes stomach juices and washes out enzymes, delaying digestion. So unless one were to chug entire liters of water between meals, the recommendation is excessive and impractical. Drinking a gallon of water *in addition to* a day's worth of calories is inferior to consuming the equivalent amount of water packed naturally in food. In other words, the recommendation is in reverse: Eighty percent of the water in the diet should derive from what we eat rather than what we drink.

How to achieve this? Glad you asked.

Emphasis should be placed on those foods whose make-up by weight is mainly water. What foods fit the bill? As a group, animal foods are low in water, as are nuts, seeds and grains. Fruits and vegetables, on the other hand, derive as much as 90 percent or more of their weight from water. Watermelons, tomatoes, lettuce, eggplant and celery, just to name a few, contain more than 90 percent water. Apples, peaches and oranges are 85 percent water. Kidney beans contain more than 75 percent water. At 95 percent, a cucumber is almost pure water. One cucumber (300 grams; 50 calories) provides more than a cup of water. Assuming an average water content for fruits and vegetables of 70 percent (an underestimation, clearly), each piece of fruit or cup of vegetables is the equivalent of 6 oz of water. Ten servings of these foods amounts to nearly 8 glasses of water, mixed with vitamins, minerals and fiber, and without even one drop drunk. Of course, 10 servings of fruits and vegetables is pretty paltry, and once you get a hang of the Paradigm, you'll find yourself consuming double this amount, with ease. In so doing, you'll notice your fiber levels approaching the limit of feasibility, and with your gut so healthy, you'll wonder how you ever ate any other way.

Back to water.

So fruits and vegetables are naturally packed in water and a diet that emphasizes these foods contains several liters of liquid. What's more, the water they contain is naturally filtered through the roots and leaves, so all the worries surrounding drinking water – the fluoride, disinfectants, pharmaceuticals, pesticides, bacteria and other contaminants – are out the window. Fruits and vegetables are also a natural source of electrolytes, including potassium. This is not to say you should avoid drinking liquid, only that beverages are meant to supplement your water intake rather than be its main source.

Recall that we suggest obtaining 20 percent of your water intake from drinking fluids. If, by the old recommendations, 80 percent is 8 to 12 glasses, then 100 percent is 10 to 15 glasses (2.5 to 3.5 L), 20 percent of which is 2 or 3 glasses, per day. (We like math, can you tell?) To fulfill this requirement, simply drink one glass of water on awakening, and one glass before lunch and before dinner, in addition to one glass before and after exercise. Because fluids can dilute the digestion, limit intake to a few oz (sips) with meals.

It is important to drink enough water to replace fluids lost during exercise. In an hour-long workout, or even just working in the heat, it is not uncommon to lose as much as 2 or 3 lbs of fluid, in the breath and sweat. In dry conditions, sweat evaporates so rapidly, you might not even know you are perspiring. Trust us, you are. An easy way to determine your fluid losses (as well as your replacement needs) is to weigh yourself before and after working out. Two lbs of weight loss equals 1 L of sweat, or about 4 cups of water.

Sweat also contains sodium. In fact, 1 L of sweat contains 1 gram of sodium, equal to 2.5 grams of sodium chloride, or table salt.[44] The recommended intake for salt in moderately active adults is 3.8 grams a day. Most people far exceed the recommended intake, in large part due to the added sodium present in packaged foods and in many restaurant meals, as well as the common propensity to dump salt over anything on a plate. Doctors warn against high salt intakes, as levels exceeding 6 grams per day are associated with high blood pressure, which in turn can lead to kidney and heart disease.[45] However, for the fitness enthusiast who derives the bulk of her calories from unprocessed foods (fruits and vegetables), adequate attention needs to be devoted not to avoiding salt, but to assuring she takes in enough. Sodium is a crucial electrolyte involved in the transmission of nervous signals. It helps regulate fluid balance and aids your body's absorption of nutrients. Therefore, take care to replace your salt losses along with your water losses. As fruits and vegetables contain minimal sodium, a convenient way to add salt to your diet is to season your evening meal. A good rule of thumb: For every liter of water you lose as sweat (2 lbs), take in an additional ½ tsp of sea salt, which contains roughly 1 g of sodium.

Remember, the planet is mostly water, and so are we. And plant foods make three.

IN SUMMARY

To reiterate, plant foods – sweets, greens, beans and seeds – best approximate, and in the case of some vegetable fruits achieve exactly, the macronutrient ratio that is most favorable to health, while being naturally high in fiber, water and micronutrients.

Is this news to you? Probably not. Everybody knows they should eat more fruits and vegetables. Moms say it, doctors urge it, teachers encourage it. And yet, too few do it! The USDA recommends five to 13 servings of fruits and vegetables a day. Less than 15 percent of Americans eat at least five. Why? Because, though most know the WHAT (fruits and vegetables) they don't know the WHY or the HOW. Knowing *how* food is handled by the digestion will help us to understand *why* the proper foods should predominate in the diet. Then we can learn *how* to go about eating more of them.

DIGESTION

If you drive a car, you may not have a clue about what goes on underneath the hood. That's fine. It is enough to fill it with gas, and when you have engine trouble, you call a mechanic. Besides, even in city traffic you likely do not spend more than a couple of hours a day behind the wheel.

But you live in your body. All day, every day. Three hundred sixty-five days each year, for a lifetime. And the body's mechanic, the doctor, knows very little of what your engine needs. In four years of medical school, the study of nutrition is limited to a few hours, if that. When as a medical student I studied pathology, we skipped over the entire chapter on nutrition. The assumption was, if doctors keep people healthy, who will fill their waiting rooms? So you cannot rely on a doctor to effectively counsel you on disease prevention, teach you how your body works or even fix you when you've broken down. Translation: You need to be the mechanic of you. So let's have a look under your hood.

The gastrointestinal tract begins with the mouth and ends with the anus. Connecting our two largest orifices is one long (30 foot) tube with four parts, which are, from proximal to distal: esophagus, stomach, small intestine and large intestine (colon).

In general, the esophagus receives food, the stomach digests it, the small intestine absorbs it and the large intestine makes waste.

Structures outside the gut but involved in digestion include the pancreas, liver and gallbladder. These organs work together to achieve the same function: to break down the food you eat into smaller molecules that the body can use.

The digestive process begins in the mouth, where the teeth mash and grind food into smaller particles. Chewing one's food is an important and often underestimated step of digestion. Thoroughly chewing food makes nutrients more available for assimilation. It increases the surface area of food morsels, a task which when you wolf down food is left to the stomach and can result in stomach upset. In addition, longer periods in the mouth allow for increased exposure to a key enzyme involved in the breakdown of starch (a type of carbohydrate). This results in improved digestion.

Your gut handles each macronutrient – protein, carbohydrate and fat – differently. Let's start with carbs.

Carbohydrates

Carbohydrate digestion begins in the mouth, where **salivary amylase** begins to break down starch before it passes through the stomach and into the small intestine. Amylase is a type of enzyme.

What are enzymes? Good question. Enzymes are protein molecules that catalyze chemical reactions. In other words, they make metabolic events in your body happen quickly and efficiently. In fact enzyme reactions occur 1,000 to 100,000,000 times faster than they otherwise would. Wow, that sure is speedy!

Enzymes are highly specific, meaning they act on one or a few substrates and catalyze only one type of chemical reaction. Digestive enzymes get released in response to food.

Salivary amylase targets dietary starch, or long chains of glucose molecules found in high quantities in the so-called *starchy* vegetables, specifically potatoes, carrots and squash. Legumes also contain large amounts of starch, as do bananas. Carbohydrate foods that do not contain starch – basically fruits and vegetables that consist of the simple sugars, fructose, glucose and sucrose – pass through the stomach unchanged and from there enter the small intestine.

In the small intestine, carbohydrate digestion continues and the simple sugars (glucose, fructose) enter the blood for use as fuel.

Fat

The bulk of fat digestion occurs in the small intestine, where pancreatic lipase (*lipo* meaning fat, as in liposuction) turns the fat in food into fatty acids to be absorbed. Because fat molecules are more complex than carbohydrates, fat sends signals to your stomach to slow emptying time, with the result that fat digestion takes longer than carbohydrate digestion. Stomach emptying is also delayed by the presence of large amounts of acid in your intestine, a consequence of eating protein-rich foods. In other words, carbohydrates are digested more rapidly than protein and fat.

Let's pause here for a moment.

So far we have touched on the digestion of carbohydrates and fats. We mentioned them in the same breath (figuratively speaking, of course) because they have something in common. The enzymes that digest starch and fat (amylase and lipase, respectively) share this characteristic: The bulk of their digestion occurs in the small intestine and both require alkaline (basic) environments. Alkaline is the opposite of acid. In other words, they don't like acid, which is probably why they don't spend much time in your stomach! In fact, these enzymes find stomach acid so inhospitable, that the pancreas releases a neutralizer (bicarbonate) so that once the stomach contents hit the small intestine, no one will get burned.

Protein

Proteins, on the other hand, love acid. In fact, they are themselves acid. Amino acids, specifically. Proteins are at home in the acidic medium of the stomach, and this is where the bulk of their digestion occurs. Not to bog ourselves down in details, but the cells of the stomach release pepsin. Pepsin is a *protease*, or protein-digesting enzyme. Enzymes are proteins, and pepsin is a protein that is activated by hydrochloric acid, which the stomach also releases. Pepsin is maximally active at a pH of 2, which is almost as acidic as it gets! Stay with us. So (stomach) acid activates protein (pepsin), which breaks down (dietary) protein into (amino) acids. The operative term here is clearly this: **ACID**. You can sometimes feel it at the back of your throat after a large protein meal. Does the word itself give you indigestion or what?

To summarize: The digestion of both carbohydrates and fats occurs mainly in the alkaline environment of the small intestine. Protein digestion takes place in the stomach in the presence of large amounts of acid, the more protein consumed, the more acid produced.

Now that we understand how each macronutrient is digested, we can infer how different foods are handled, depending on which nutrient predominates.

Fruit

Fruit is primarily simple sugars, the sweeter the fruit the simpler the sugars. Grapes, for example, are 95 percent carbohydrate, and of this, 98.7 percent consists of equal amounts of free glucose and free fructose. These simple sugars enter the mouth essentially predigested. In other words, they require no digestive enzymes to break them down. They quickly pass through your stomach and into your small intestine, where they are rapidly absorbed to provide instant energy. Because of its rapid digestibility, fruit is best eaten alone. Otherwise it interferes with the digestion of other foods, while its own digestion is retarded. (As with most things in life, your digestion is only as fast as its slowest link.) It is therefore best to consume fruit *on its own*.

Vegetables and Legumes

Vegetables and legumes (beans, peas, lentils) are starchier than fruits. The long chains of sugars present in most vegetables and beans require the work of several enzymes (amylase, maltase, sucrase, to name them). But vegetables are mostly water and fiber, which assist the digestion in the breakdown of these molecules. Though these foods leave the stomach more slowly than fruits, the body can effectively break them down in a fraction of the time required by more concentrated foods such as nuts, grains, meat and dairy. These foods lack water and fiber and instead contain lots of fat, which slows stomach emptying (remember?), and/or protein, which sits in the stomach for long periods while enzymes break it down.

Grains

Grains are starchier and more concentrated than vegetables including beans. Brown rice, for instance, has twice the starch and 30 percent more calories than kidney beans. To assimilate all this starch, the pancreas must secrete a large quantity of amylase, which over time can lead to burnout!

Meat, Eggs, Dairy

Animal products, being predominately protein, remain in the stomach for long periods and in contrast to starchy grains (and fats) require an acid medium. The more protein eaten, the more acid is secreted. The high stomach acidity that occurs when proteins are ingested increases when proteins are broken down into amino acids, which as we said are acids themselves.

Most animal products also contain a generous percentage of fat. Remember, fat digestion occurs in the small intestine, not in the stomach, as is the case with protein. It's as if meat wanted to be in two places at once! Of course, this is not possible, as anyone who ever wanted to be in bed sleeping while taking an hour-long exam at school can attest.

As you might have predicted, the protein-induced acid release slows the digestion of fat. In some cases, extreme acidification can inactivate lipase, the enzyme that digests fat. As a result, dietary fats are not adequately digested or absorbed, and fat is excreted in the stool. This condition is known as steatorrhea and is characterized by greasy, frothy stools that float. (We hope you're not reading this over dinner!)

For this reason, to combine protein and fat, either separately as in chicken fried in oil, or a pepperoni pizza, or together in the same food - remember, meat, eggs and dairy derive most or all of their calories from a combination of protein and fat - is to wreak havoc on your insides. The result is not digestion but congestion (stuffy, anyone?) and fatigue.

It would seem from this that animal products are not our preferred food.

To make matters worse, these same foods, lacking water and fiber, are concentrated foods. Each mouthful of meat, or peanut butter, or scrambled eggs, or ice cream, brings with it more calories, and consequently involves more digestive effort, than the same-sized bite of fruits or vegetables.

The digestive fiasco caused by combining proteins and fat also occurs when starches (bread, pasta, cereal) are combined with proteins (meat, cheese). As with fats, grains cannot be broken down until the acidity required by protein digestion has been reduced. *The show simply will not go on!* What results is a battle between the stomach and its hydrochloric acid, versus the pancreas and its alkaline neutralizer. Like cars stuck at an intersection whose stoplight is rapidly alternating between red and green, improperly combined food has nowhere to go. It lingers in the stomach and ferments (in the case of fruit) or turns rancid (fats), or putrefies, as is the case with protein. This could lead to all types of accidents. Crash!

What are the symptoms of this catastrophe? The result of excess acid is heartburn. Foods lacking in fiber cause constipation. Incompletely digested food, rushed by injudicious combination with fruit, makes its way into the large intestine where bacteria metabolize it into hydrogen and methane, causing flatulence (farts, yuck!). Consequently, after a meal of say, spaghetti with meat sauce, and apple pie for dessert, the dinner guest is left bloated, backed-up and burping up stomach acid, and in no mood to dance.

To reiterate, poorly combined foods and too many concentrated foods fester in the stomach for much longer than they otherwise would, and/or are rushed through the small intestine before being completely assimilated. Their energy (if they contain any, and meat, which is zero carbohydrate, does not) is prevented from entering the bloodstream; moreover, so much enzymatic activity is required to break down such foods, that by eating them, one is essentially depleting his energy stores instead of adding to them. This is why the predominant feeling after eating things foods such as pizza, or hamburgers, or breakfast cereal with milk, is fatigue. In fact, most dietary staples are examples of poorly-combined, concentrated foods that spell disaster for the digestion and are lessons in what NOT to do.

WHAT NOT TO DO

Chicken wrap: starch (tortilla) combined with protein (poor food combination); where's the water? (too concentrated)

Pepperoni pizza: starch (bread), protein (meat), fat (cheese); too concentrated

Sushi: starch (rice) and protein (fish); too concentrated

Bean and rice burrito: rice on beans on flour is too much starch

Trail mix: poor food combination (fruit with nuts)

Breakfast cereal with milk: protein (milk) and starch (grains); too concentrated

Peanut butter sandwich: too concentrated (grain and nut); poor food combining (if jelly is used)

Not to get too anthropological on you (yet!), but if you analyze our evolution as a species, you'll find that before the Agricultural Revolution 10,000 years ago, before we began eating milk products and eggs (6,000 years ago), before meat, before even cooked food, our natural inclinations as well as environmental conditions led us to encounter quantities of a particular fruit or vegetable, say in a strawberry patch or field of greens, and to devour this food until our senses were indulged and our metabolic needs met. Our body is designed to handle one type of food at a time, or more practically, one food group. To saddle ourselves with so many different foods, so many different ingredients, is to ask for disaster. Next time you pick up that packaged food (which we hope will be the last) note the long list of ingredients, which often runs the length of a paragraph, and ask yourself: Was I really designed to take in all this *stuff* at once, if at all? One word: Not!

What about plant foods? Although fruits and vegetables contain a proportion of all calorie types, they are mostly water, carbohydrates and fiber, in that order, with on average only minimal (5 to 10 percent) protein or fat, and are handled as such, either on their own or eaten together, with relative ease.

To illustrate: Take 1 small apple, which weighs 100 grams and provides 50 calories. Eighty-five and a half grams is in the form of water and 2.5 grams is fiber. In other words 88 percent of an apple, by weight, is calorie-free. No digestion is involved. No effort required, no enzymes needed. It's just packaging, helping to deliver the nutrients to your cells and the toxins out your bottom. The remaining 12 grams is almost entirely (96 percent, or 11.5 grams) carbohydrate, with only .5 grams in the form of protein and fat.

Even spinach, which derives nearly half of its calories from protein, is so high in water and fiber that it is virtually impossible to take in large quantities of protein from spinach without stuffing oneself. To eat a mere 100 calories of raw baby spinach, you'd have to serve yourself 20 cups! Go see if you can find a big enough bowl to accommodate that amount of bulk!

By contrast, let's look at nuts, which are one of the driest foods on the planet. A 100 gram serving of walnuts, equal to 4 oz, contains a total of 10 grams of water and fiber, combined. That's only 10 percent, by weight, in contrast to an apple's 90 percent. The remaining 90 percent of weight in walnuts is mainly fat (65 grams) and a protein/carbohydrate mix (22 grams). A lot of digestive effort goes into metabolizing the over 650 calories that 100 grams of walnuts contains. Lots of lipase, lots of amylase, lots of protease. Do nuts give you energy? They seem to require more than they are worth. Why saddle yourself with this dead weight?

Instead, eat sweets, greens, beans and seeds. Then, repeat.

WHAT TO DO

1. Fruit on its own for breakfast. It's easy to digest and rapidly absorbed to provide instant energy. Eating fresh fruit on its own through lunch is also an option. Dinner might include a mixture of beans and vegetables (raw and lightly-cooked).

2. Fresh fruit for lunch, and/or a large raw salad.

3. Two or three vegetable dishes for dinner, with beans and/or potatoes.

4. Fruit for dessert, if desired.

IN SUMMARY

Since different foods are handled differently by the digestion, and appropriate enzymes require time to re-accumulate, wait a minimum of 3 hours between plant-based meals, or more than 4 hours if the meal includes animal products or other concentrated foods. This helps to ensure the stomach is empty and enzymes are restored. Fruit is of course the exception. Eat fruit on its own throughout the day. If taken with vegetables, fruit may cause stomach upset. It is better to wait for some time between consuming the two rather than to combine them, but if you must eat fruits and vegetables together, *eat them raw*, preferably blended in a shake.

It is best to avoid all concentrated foods, which are, once again: nuts, grains, meat, eggs and dairy.

Now, you may be asking, does food combination really matter? If every food has a combination of all three macronutrients, doesn't combining foods just add more to the mix? To a certain degree, this is correct. For example, take mixing raisins with sweet potatoes. Although it does taste delicious, mixing fruit with vegetable is not perfect food combining. Remember, fruit is so rapidly digested that it is best to consume fruit on its own. And yet, since the sugar in raisin complements the starch in sweet potatoes, the nutrient breakdown of this delicious combination is very similar to eating bananas, which are high in both starch and simple sugars.

<u>1 Medium Sweet Potato and 1 Miniature Box of Raisins</u>
132 calories
2.43 g protein
.21 g fat
31 g carbohydrate
3.8 g fiber
14.77 g total sugars
7.43 g starch

vs.

<u>1 Extra Large Banana</u>
135 calories
1.66 g protein
.5 g fat

34.75 g carbohydrate
4 g fiber
18.6 g total sugars
8.2 g starch

Eating bananas is certainly nutritious. If the nutrient break-down is the same, why could mixing raisins and sweet potato be any different? You are catching on. These foods are nutritious, alone or combined. High in water and fiber, they are easy to digest. Eat them to your heart's content.

The problem occurs when you combine large quantities of concentrated foods that have drastic differences in their nutrient profiles: say, starch with protein, or protein with fat. The effect is to overwhelm your digestive capacities and the result is indigestion. Bottom line: Don't do it!

For example, eating a tuna fish sandwich provides 320 calories, 42 grams of protein and 23 grams of starch, which places a heavy toll on your digestive enzymes (amylases and proteases, among others) and can only result in fatigue and burnout. A slice of meat pizza is another example. Ten grams of protein, 12 grams of fat, 28 grams of carbohydrate, about 1 gram of fiber and 1 oz of water. Disaster waiting to happen. Please don't.

ABSORPTION

Once digested, macronutrients enter the bloodstream. Carbohydrates, fats and proteins all converge at a point in your metabolism called the TCA cycle. At this point, what is left is a two-carbon molecule called acetyl-CoA (there's a five dollar word to impress your friends). The process is pretty complex, so here's the gist: With the help of oxygen from your lungs, acetyl-CoA becomes carbon dioxide while forming adenosine triphosphate, or ATP. ATP is the energy currency of your cells.

Carbs, protein, fat ------> acetyl CoA -------> ATP

Wait, I thought you said carbohydrates are energy!

Yes carbohydrate is your body's preferred fuel, and glucose swims in your blood, but in order to be used, carbs (and fats, and proteins) must first form ATP.

ATP. Energy. Say it again. It rhymes!

For example, one molecule of glucose yields 36 ATPs. That's a lot of ATP/energy! Fatty acids yield even more, roughly 131 ATPs per molecule. By contrast, only some amino acids can make energy. These *glucogenic* amino acids, as they are called, yield a relatively small amount of ATP. This is another reason a common side effect of high protein diets is fatigue.

ELIMINATION

Waste products, aided by water and fiber, pass through the colon and are eliminated as stool. With few exceptions, bowel regularity can be seen as a reflection of fiber intake. The more fiber in the diet, the greater the frequency and the bulk of bowel movements.

Plant foods, bulkier and with more fiber and water, encourage both the *gastrocolic reflex* and a phenomenon known as *peristalsis*, or contractions of the bowels, which lead to swifter passage through the colon.

Animal products, in contrast, can fester in the gut for several days, giving rise to foul-smelling, hard, pebbly stool, and setting the stage for constipation, hemorrhoids, even anal fissures. Sensitive individuals, such as those with milk intolerance or food allergies, may experience just the opposite: stomach cramps, offensive flatulence and explosive diarrhea.

Bowel transit time refers to how long it takes for food to move through you, measured from the moment you munch it in to the time you pinch it out.

Munch-pinch. Say it again. Munch-pinch. Say it loud. MUNCH-PINCH!

Normal transit time is between 36 and 48 hours. Longer than 72 hours is considered sluggish.[46] How do you measure up? To determine the length of time it takes for food to go from your mouth to your anus, you could perform a little experiment at home: Eat something with a distinctive color, such as beets, and over the next few days observe your stool until you no longer see red. Or to get a ballpark figure, you could answer this simple question: meat or no meat?

We know that bowel transit time is influenced by the amount of fiber in the diet, with intakes of greater than 30 g being associated with more rapid transit, and since vegetarians generally eat more fiber than meat eaters, you can determine your transit time just by falling into one or the other group: carnivore or herbivore.

In one famous study,[47] vegetarian males were found to have transit times up to 60 hours, which is less than the 72-hour limit, but still seems kind of long. Who knows, maybe these dudes ate a lot of cheese? But the vegetarian times seem like a blink of an eye compared to the meat-eaters, who took up to 132 hours to evacuate their bowels. That is 5 ½ days from trap to shoot. Talk about backed up!

In other words, if you indulge in flesh, chances are the steak sandwich you have on Sunday evening won't be going *kerplunk* until next Friday night, at which time it will probably be smelling pretty darn foul. Who knows, maybe you'll happen to be at a party, in which case it'd be called *party foul!*

Toilet humor aside, while we're on the subject of poop, let's ask the question: What constitutes bowel regularity? In other words, how often should you, you know, go? Hopefully more than once a week, but how often exactly? As with most things in the medical profession, the answer depends on whom you ask. So let's use our old friend common sense. For our answer, likely the right one, we have only to look at infants, whose digestive systems are in perfect working order. They're cute, they're cuddly, and they poop a lot! In general, infants pass stool after every feeding. This should be seen as our model through adulthood and into old age (or the golden years, if you prefer). Anything less than several bulky stools per diem reflects problematic digestion likely due to poor food combining or to the wrong foods altogether (or more likely, to both) and deserves the term constipation.

Three poops per day? you say. Yes, preferably all in the AM.

What does your stool say about you? Is your poop pencil thin? Is it greasy or frothy? Does it float on the water's surface? Is it pebbly? Is it so watery that it splashes and sprays the toilet rim? How about black and tarry? Clay-colored? With chunks of undigested food? Blood-tinged or mucus streaked? If your bowel movements resemble any of these characteristic types, which are all pathologic, your digestion is in disarray. Stool should be soft and of the size and shape of an extra large banana. To produce bananas from your bowels, focus on fruit. You are what you eat, and so is your poop.

TAKE THIS TO THE TABLE

Eat fruit on its own for breakfast.

Make fruits and vegetables a major part, if not the only part, of lunch and dinner.

Chew each mouthful a minimum of 20 times.

Make each meal last 20 minutes or longer. To slow down, eat with family and friends. Use chopsticks.

Wait a minimum of 3 hours between meals, or 30 minutes after eating fruit before consuming other foods.

Minimize or eliminate concentrated foods (meat, eggs, dairy, grains and nuts).

Now, you can take our word for it and follow these rules, but few people (including us) like to be told what to do. So, if you need more convincing that not all calories are created equal and some give you instant energy and move rapidly through you while others drop like a lead load into your gut and require tremendous effort to digest, you may wish to conduct an energy experiment on yourself. Try this.

For the next 7 days, eat this for breakfast. On each day, you'll be consuming a 500-calorie meal from each of the major food groups.

Day One: 8 medium oranges
Day Two: 5 cups of steamed broccoli
Day Three: 2.5 cups of garbanzo beans
Day Four: 5 slices of cheese
Day Five: 3 oz peanuts
Day Six: 2.5 cups cooked spaghetti
Day Seven: 2.5 cans of tuna

After each meal, take note of how you feel for the remainder of the day. How is your energy level? What's your appetite for lunch and dinner like? How are your bowel movements? How thirsty are you?

Then, rank each of the 7 meals in terms of enjoyment, energy and whether or not you'd be likely to eat it again. We have a feeling day one will be Number One.

MICRONUTRIENTS

Vitamins and minerals are the **micronutrients**. Why *micro*? Because you need less of these in your diet than the macronutrients. As we saw, macronutrient intake is measured in grams per day, while the daily requirement of most micronutrients is in milligrams, or one thousandth of a gram. For some vitamins, such as vitamin B12, intakes are in micrograms. One microgram is one thousandth of a milligram, or one millionth of a gram. Very tiny indeed, but nonetheless super important. Why? Because your body cannot synthesize most vitamins and minerals and so you must obtain them in your diet, as we have seen is the case with the essential amino acids.

Just as all carbohydrate derives from the sun, and all protein originates from green vegetation, many vitamins and minerals ascend to us from the soil, where they are present naturally as part of the Earth or are synthesized by microorganisms (bacteria).

Among the micronutrients are the antioxidants (vitamins A, C, E and the mineral selenium). You've probably heard of them. Antioxidants protect the body from damage caused by free radicals, which are highly reactive derivatives of oxygen. Hydrogen peroxide is one example. No, not the kind you buy at the drug store, although the chemical formula is the same: H_2O_2. Free radicals are formed continuously within the body. They occur as by-products of metabolism, through reactions with drugs, dietary and environmental toxins, and when levels of antioxidants get too low. Excessive amounts of free radicals contribute to cancer, heart disease and premature aging.[48] So where do antioxidants come in? Glad you asked. Antioxidants neutralize free radicals, which is why maintaining a steady intake of them is important. What are the major sources of antioxidants? Fruits and vegetables, almost exclusively.

Like water and fiber, vitamins and minerals are calorie-free, yet they are part of every calorie that is nutritious.

Okay, I get it, you may be saying. *Vitamins and minerals are important. Are you really going to make me memorize them?*

Really, there is no reason – unless you go to medical school, in which case you will have to, to do good on tests. There are over 20 essential vitamins and minerals. Added to this are the thousands of identified phytonutrients (*phyto* = plant) and most likely many more that haven't been discovered. To analyze each individual nutrient or try and link *this* food with *that* vitamin or *that* mineral with *this* health benefit is futile and quickly becomes frustrating. (Unless you make a song from it: "It's like this and like that and like this and..." Uh, that's already been done.) Besides, we're not in med school anymore, and we're not trying to sell you any supplements.

Can we just infer that plant foods, being higher in water and fiber and containing a proper mix of the macronutrients, are most likely highest in the other nutrients and from there just move on to their preparation?

Perhaps for evidence we could simply consult authorities in history and anthropology, determine from them the diets that sustained our ancestors for thousands upon thousands of years and just follow their lead. Indeed, anthropological evidence supports the consumption of predominately plants, but the average diet has drastically changed in the 6 million years since our ancestors divided from the chimpanzees. For much of this time, our food grew from the Earth and was gathered and eaten raw. And chimpanzees, who share 95 percent of our DNA, have remained loyal to this diet, eating over 50 percent fruit. Yes, you read that correctly. Over half of the primate diet is devoted to sweet fruit, as the breakthrough research conducted by paleoanthropologist Jane Goodall has shown, with the remainder derived mainly from leafy green vegetables, a small portion of seeds, and perhaps and insect or two. (And the occasional pig. It is true that chimps infrequently engage in hunting; however, meat accounts for under 5 percent of the primate diet and shouldn't be viewed as an example of what to do but rather of what NOT to do. After all, chimps are animals, while humans should aspire to transcend our bestial nature and approach the divine. Don't you think?)

From our plant-based origins we have evolved (or *de*volved) to experiment with many diets. In the 150,000 that *homo sapiens* have been around, we have foraged, plucked, gathered, caught, killed, cooked, seasoned, dehydrated, denatured, refried, fortified, mass-produced, packaged, processed, chemically-engineered and genetically-modified our food, so that most of what we now eat bears little resemblance to the whole food from which it derived.

Some anthropologists view meat eating as part of the evolutionary step that led to an increase in the size of the human brain. The theory is that because meat provides more concentrated calories than vegetation, by eating meat our ancestors were for the first time able to meet their caloric needs, and to grow.

Other scholars view it the other way around: Meat eating, they say, came after an increase in brain size. With bigger brains came more effective tools, which made for successful hunting. The brain enlargement, they say, was due to a diet of nutrient-rich plants. According to these experts, meat, which contains far fewer vitamins and minerals than the plants from which it ultimately derives, should be viewed as a *de*volutionary step. In other words, we evolved *because of* plant foods and *despite* animal food consumption.

Both sides agree, however, that whatever its effect on brain size, due to its large proportion of saturated fat and concentrated calories, and the relatively sedentary existence of modern humans, one body part that meat eating most definitely enlarges in today's world, is the belly...and maybe the buttocks.

One could make a very convincing argument that since animals built like us (gorillas and other primates) eat fruits and vegetables and very little fat or animal products, so should we. That, since the biggest, strongest animals (elephants and rhinoceroses, for instance) and many of the fastest (antelope, gazelle) all eat predominately green vegetation, these foods can certainly build our muscles and meet our needs. Or that our gastrointestinal anatomy argues in favor of fruit and vegetable consumption and against the consumption of meat.

There are many differences in the anatomies of humans and carnivores. Take your dog, for instance. Dogs are true carnivores, with a digestive system suited to meat. Dogs have a rasping tongue for lopping up blood; our tongues are smooth. Dogs have claws to rip through muscle; we do not. Our molars are flat, whereas the sharp incisors of man's best friend are ideal for tearing apart flesh. The salivary pH of the dog is acidic while ours is more alkaline. This allows dogs to easily digest the protein in meat and tolerate the bacteria present in rotting flesh, while our pH is more suited to carbohydrate foods and indeed contains the enzyme amylase, which breaks down plant starch.

There are other differences. The human bowel is convoluted and measuring 30 feet is over ten times the length of our torso, with pouches; the bowels of carnivores are built like chimney stacks, short and straight. As a result, food passes through the carnivore much more quickly; they can easily handle the cholesterol, fat and chemicals in animal foods and have much less need for fiber. In humans, meat festers in the pouches and clings to bowel walls; the digestion of meat produces cancer-causing substances. In fact, the feces of a meat eater and those of a plant eater can be distinguished on the basis of smell, with the former being foul-smelling, which indicates the presence of putrefying flesh. Plant poop, by contrast, is odor-free.

Does it suffice to say that only the food which, in its natural state - raw, unseasoned and unrefined - causes us to salivate and fills us with longing is fit for our consumption, while whatever in its natural state causes disgust, revulsion or any emotion other than joy and desire should be avoided? (If given the choice between a cherry tree and a cow at pasture, to which would you turn to satisfy hunger?)

There are those who advocate what is known as a Paleolithic approach to the diet, which involves eating what cavemen may have eaten thousands of years ago: meat, nuts and relatively little vegetation or fruits.

The proponents of such a dietary approach argue that from 2.5 million years ago until the start of the Agricultural Revolution, or Neolithic Period, humans ate a largely animal-based diet. They argue that the human digestive system has not evolved to handle grains and dairy products, which were introduced into the diet 10,000 years ago and to which they attribute a variety of modern ailments such as diabetes, high blood pressure and heart disease, the so-called diseases of affluence. We agree: Grains and dairy products are bad for our health. But does this mean we're meant to digest meat?

Let us go back in time before the Paleolithic Era. Before then, we had no stone tools. The sharp canine teeth had been lost to our species by at least three and a half million years ago. During the million years up until the invention of tools, what did we eat? A great deal of uncooked plants. Like cattle, horses and other natural vegetarians, we have molars for crushing food rather than knife-like incisors for cutting through flesh. Without the restriction of large canine teeth, our jaws are able to move somewhat side-to-side, making them ideally suited to crushing vegetation.

And so, 3.5 million years ago, we lost our canine teeth, and with them, our meat-eating propensities. This was the true evolutionary step. One million years later, with the invention of stone tools our ancestors reverted to the consumption of animal flesh, which should be viewed as taking a step backwards.

Some may imagine that we resumed flesh eating as hunters, but according to paleoanthropologist Dr. Richard Leakey, this is simply not the case. In a desperate search for calories, humans ate what they could find, and with tools to tear flesh, this did include animal tissue. But unlike the true predators, lions and tigers, early humans had trouble catching and killing prey on their own and were lucky to find the left-overs of real predators. In other words, we scrambled for scraps. We scavenged for sloppy seconds, if you will. Our ancestors were more like coyotes, hyenas or the particularly unbecoming jackal, except for one major difference: These scavengers are true carnivores, with digestions suited to flesh.

Ours is anything but.

For us, including animal flesh in the diet was (and is) not without its dangers. Humans cannot handle the fat and cholesterol of meat, which is the true cause of the variety of modern ailments and Western diseases on which the "Paleo" followers blame grains, dairy and processed sugars. By contrast, it is impossible to give carnivores (dogs, for example) high cholesterol, even by feeding them great quantities of butter! Why? Because carnivores are designed to consume animal foods, taking what they need and eliminating the toxins and other harmful chemicals. On the other hand, giving a herbivore (say, rabbits) cholesterol produces striking changes in the arterial wall, similar to the atherosclerotic plaques seen in humans.[49]

It would seem wise therefore to learn the lessons of history and understand the design of our digestive anatomy, leaving the scraps to the hyenas and concerning ourselves with crushing nutrient-rich plants.

If this evolutionary argument against including animal products in your diet does not satisfy, one might raise the point that our cavemen ancestors included human flesh in their dietary preferences. That's right, between grunts and groans, the parents of our race were cannibals.[50] Does this mean modern humans should devour each other like savages? Come to think of it, we already do. With modern artillery and other engines of war, we decimate populations, slaughtering our neighbors and endangering the future of the human race, which merits a discussion of its own.

But should we actually consume each others' flesh, just because prehistoric humans did? Of course not. So why should we, at this advanced stage of human evolution, persist in the habits of our genetic infancy and continue in a practice so backwards as flesh eating? As babies we all wore diapers. Does this mean adults should walk around in Pampers and Huggies, crying goo-goo and gaa-gaa? Please.

Need we mention that Neanderthals were also predominately meat eaters only to fall into extinction? Perhaps we should learn the lessons of history and realize that endangering the lives of other species by consuming them for food endangers our own. Eating meat was born from necessity. In times of famine, animal flesh provided a concentrated source of calories and enabled our ancestors to survive long winters without much food. We now live in a time of plenty, and meat eating no longer serves an evolutionary purpose. In fact, the environmental hazards of eating meat are so horrific that if the practice is allowed to continue it may bring about the famines of ancient times, as we shall explore later on.

Back to our discussion.

Though these arguments may appeal to logic, intuition and common sense, they don't stand up to the scrutiny of the scientist, who doggedly, if a bit cynically, requires facts and facts alone. Fortunately, scientific discoveries have finally caught up with human evolution, proving that the diet that has nourished the human race for the bulk of its existence is also far and away the maximally nutritious.

NUTRIENT DENSITY

Medical experts have devised rating systems that assign values to foods based on their nutrient density. The nutrient density of a food is determined by the proportion of essential vitamins and minerals and known phytonutrients, to calories. The higher the proportion, the more nutrients per calorie, the higher the nutrient density, and the higher the score.

How do various foods fare? Leafy green vegetables score highest. Spinach, kale and Romaine lettuce, for example, get a perfect score of 100. Then come solid green vegetables (score: 95), followed by other non-starchy vegetables, beans and fresh fruits, which receive a strong score of 50.

From there scores drop precipitously. The other *traditional* food groups (grains, meat, eggs, fish, dairy, nuts and refined foods) all score a measly 20 or below, and in some cases the already low values assigned to these nutritionally inferior foods may in fact be an over-estimation of their nutritiousness.

You see, the nutrient density scoring system does not take into consideration the toxic elements in food. In other words, it evaluates foods based on their nutrients (vitamins and minerals) not their anti-nutrients (saturated fat, cholesterol and oxidants, for example). As most of the nutrient-deficient foods (animal foods and re-fined foods) also happen to contain a large proportion of anti-nutrients, their scores could justifiably be much lower, so that the flimsy 5 that cheese scores, when you consider the lack of fiber in cheese coupled with its high levels of saturated fat, cholesterol, antibiotics, hormones, pesticides and fertilizer residues, is actually much closer to zero.

DENSITY SCORES[51]

95-100	Green vegetables
50	Non-starchy vegetables, legumes, fruits
35	Starchy vegetables (potatoes and squash)
20	Whole grains, nuts
15 (0)	Fish, fat-free dairy
10 (0)	Meat, eggs
5 (0)	Cheese
1 (0)	Refined grains, oils, sweets

You have heard of the five major food groups. There really is only one, and it is plants.

Plants.

Unrefined, unprocessed and whole.

Plants.

To further prove the point that plants are the maximally nutritious foods, we can compare the above food groups for ourselves. Using the USDA's National Nutrient Database for Standard Reference (www.nal.usda.gov/fnic/foodcomp/search/) we can take the most nutritious food from each group, as determined by the Aggregate Nutrient Density Index (ANDI)[52], and compare them for 5 key nutrients – vitamin A, vitamin C, iron, calcium and fiber. Then, taking the average percent value for each food, we can see how they match up. To be more precise, we'll also include the number of other essential nutrients contained in significant amounts (25 percent or more of the recommended daily value).

Bear in mind that scientists also factor in ORAC scores - ORAC stands for Oxygen Radical Absorbance Capacity, a measurement of a food's antioxidant capability - and other known phytonutrients. Phytonutrients appear exclusively in plants; therefore, since we are excluding them from our simplified analysis, we are underestimating the nutritive value of fruits, vegetables and beans. Our informal comparison is not as comprehensive as the methods scientists use, but it is a very useful exercise in food analysis, one we hope you will soon repeat for meals of your very own.

Here is how the food groups measure up.

TALE OF THE TASTE

Leafy green vegetable: Spinach

calories: 100 (2.5 cups boiled)

macronutrients (in grams)

carbohydrate: 17

protein: 13.5

fat: 1

ratio (carbohydrate/protein/fat): 60-30-10

fiber: 10.8 (43% DV)

water: 14 oz

micronutrients (as %DV)

vitamin A: 943

vitamin C: 74

calcium: 61

iron: 89

Score: <u>242</u> (Average percent daily value for vitamin A, C, iron, calcium and fiber.)

Spinach also contains 25 percent or more of the DV of thiamin, B6, phosphorus, vitamin E, riboflavin, manganese, copper and magnesium.

Vegetable fruit: Red pepper

calories: 100, (2.5 cups chopped, or 2 large fruits)

macronutrients (in grams)

carbohydrate: 23

protein: 4

fat: 1

ratio: 80-10-10

fiber: 8 (32%)

water: 12 oz

micronutrients (as %DV)

vitamin A: 243

vitamin C: 825

calcium: 3

iron: 9

Score: 222

Contains 25% or more DV of B6, vitamin E

Solid green vegetable: Broccoli

calories: 100, (3 1/3 cups raw)

macronutrients (in grams)

carbohydrate: 19

protein: 8

fat: 1

ratio: 70-20-10

fiber: 7.6 (30%)

water: 8 oz

micronutrients (as %DV)

vitamin A: 36

vitamin C: 432

calcium: 14

iron: 12

Score: 105

Contains 25% or more DV of B6, manganese

Starchy vegetable: Sweet potato

calories: 100, (1 cup raw, or 1 medium)

macronutrients (in grams)

carbohydrate: 23

protein: 2

fat: 0

ratio: 92-8-0

fiber: 4 (16%)

water: 3 oz

micronutrients (as %DV)

vitamin A: 377

vitamin C: 5

calcium: 4

iron: 5

Score: 81.4

Contains 25% or more DV of no other nutrients

Other vegetable: Cauliflower

calories: 100, (4 cups raw, or ½ large head)

macronutrients (in grams)

carbohydrate: 21

protein: 8

fat: 0.5

ratio: 77-20-3

fiber: 10 (40%)

water: 12 oz

micronutrients (as %DV)

vitamin A: 1

vitamin C: 309

calcium: 9

iron: 10

Score: 74

Contains 25% or more DV of B6, manganese

Strawberry (a true fruit)

calories: 100, (2 cups, or 16 large)

<u>macronutrients (in grams)</u>

carbohydrate: 23

protein: 2

fat: 1

ratio: 85-7-8

fiber: 6 (24%)

water: 9 oz

<u>micronutrients (as %DV)</u>

vitamin A: 1

vitamin C: 298

calcium: 5

iron: 7

Score: <u>67</u>

Includes 25% or more DV of manganese

Bean: Bean sprouts (mung or soy)

calories: 100, (3 1/3 cups)

macronutrients (in grams)

carbohydrate: 20

protein: 10

fat: .5

ratio: 70-25-5

fiber: 6 (24%)

water: 10.5 oz

micronutrients (as %DV)

vitamin A: 1

vitamin C: 73

calcium: 4

iron: 17

Score: 24

Includes 25% or more DV of B6, manganese, riboflavin, copper

Dairy: Skim milk

calories: 100, (1.2 cups)

<u>macronutrients (in grams)</u>

carbohydrate: 14

protein: 10

fat: .5

ratio: 53-42-5

fiber: 0 (0%)

water: 9 oz

<u>micronutrients (as %DV)</u>

vitamin A: 0

vitamin C: 5

calcium: 35

iron: 1

Score: <u>8.2</u>

Includes 25% or more DV of phosphorus

Whole grain: Oats

calories: 100, (1/3 cup dry)

macronutrients (in grams)

carbohydrate: 18

protein: 3.5

fat: 2

ratio: 70-14-16

fiber: 2.5 (10%)

water: 0

micronutrients (as %DV)

vitamin A: 0

vitamin C: 0

calcium: 1

iron: 7

Score: 3.6

Includes 25% or more DV of manganese

Eggs

calories: 100, (1 jumbo, raw)

<u>macronutrients (in grams)</u>

carbohydrate: 0

protein: 8

fat: 6.5

ratio: 0-35-65

fiber: 0 (0%)

water: 1.5 oz

<u>micronutrients (as %DV)</u>

vitamin A: 6

vitamin C: 0

calcium: 3

iron: 7

Score: <u>3.2</u>

Includes 25% or more DV of selenium

Raw nuts: Brazil nuts

calories: 100 (0.5 oz, about 4 nuts)

macronutrients (in grams)

carbohydrates: 2

protein: 2

fat: 10

ratio: 8-8-84

fiber: 1.2 (5%)

water: 1 oz

micronutrients (as %DV)

vitamin A: 0

vitamin C: 0

calcium: 2

iron: 5

Score: 2.4

Includes 25% or more of copper, selenium

Meat: Skinless chicken breast

calories: 100, (2 oz, less than 1/3 of one small breast)

macronutrients (in mg)

carbohydrate: 0

protein: 19

fat: 2

ratio: 0-80-20

fiber: 0 (0%)

water: 1 oz

micronutrients (as %DV)

vitamin A: 0

vitamin C: 0

calcium: 1

iron: 8

Score: 1.8

Includes: 25% or more DV of B6, niacin, selenium

Fish: Tuna

calories: 100, (2.5 oz, cooked)

macronutrients (in grams)

carbohydrate: 4

protein: 8.5

fat: 3

ratio: 0-92-8

fiber: 0 (0%)

water: 1.5 oz

micronutrients (as %DV)

vitamin A: 1

vitamin C: 1

calcium: 2

iron: 4

Score: 1.6

Includes 25% or more DV of thiamin, niacin, vitamin B6

Refined grain, oils, and sweets: Olive oil

calories: 100, (less than 1 tbsp)

macronutrients (in grams)

carbohydrate: 0

protein: 0

fat: 11

ratio: 0-0-100

fiber: 0 (0%)

water: 0

micronutrients (as %DV)

vitamin A: 0

vitamin C: 0

calcium: 0

iron: 0

Score: 0

Olive oil contains no essential nutrients.

THE SCORES

The Best

Spinach: 242

Red pepper: 222

Broccoli: 105

Sweet potato: 81

Cauliflower: 74

Strawberry: 67

Bean sprouts: 24

The Rest

Skim milk: 8.2

Oats: 3.6

Eggs: 3.2

Nuts: 2.4

Chicken: 1.8

Fish:1.6

Oil: 0

As predicted, our analysis reveals that the foods with the highest nutritional value are all plants. Plant foods are without question the Paradigm foods.

The few nutrients present in high amounts in animal products — namely phosphorus, selenium, zinc and some B-vitamins — originate in plants. Remember, animals can't make most micronutrients and so must obtain them in foods, just like us. And most animals eat plants. The cow eats grass. The horse eats hay. The lion dines on the deer, which has formed its muscle from the protein found in vegetation. The sardine eats plankton. The salmon eats the sardine. Why humans regard salmon and other carnivorous fish, which are so far removed from the energy source (sun, greens) as a health food defies logic! Remember the energy ladder: sun, soil, greens/fruits, animals. The closer you remain to the ultimate energy source, the sun, the more energy you have, and the more nutrients too. And the closest we can come to eating the sun is to eat the plants that convert its glorious rays into green leaves, sweets, beans and seeds. Got it? Good!

Now, the message to eat your fruits and vegetables is by no means new. There is almost universal agreement among doctors, nutritionists and laypeople that the Paradigm foods should comprise the bulk of the diet, and many experts suggest that the nutritionally inferior foods (grains, nuts, meat, eggs, dairy, sweets, oils) be eaten in moderation *if at all*. The only organizations that oppose this view are those, such as the beef, egg and dairy industries, with vested interests in the inferior foods.

But if maximal nutrient density is the goal, and optimal health achieved, it is best to consume fruits, vegetables and beans. Exclusively, and in unlimited quantities.

Imagine a new food pyramid, with one word filling the center.

PLANTS

Next, draw another pyramid, divided in three equal parts, with SWEETS and GREENS (and other vegetables) at its base, and BEANS (and maybe some SEEDS) at its apex. Then, divide your caloric consumption between these maximally nutritious foods, and you'll reach the peak of nutrition.

SEEDS
BEANS
SWEETS
GREENS

THE PARADIGM FOODS

Sweets: apples, apricots, bananas, blackberries, blueberries, cantaloupe, cherries, dates, figs, grapefruit, grapes, lemons, limes, kiwi, mango, nectarines, melons, oranges, papayas, peaches, pears, persimmons, pineapples, plums, prunes, raisins, raspberries, strawberries, tangerines, watermelons

Greens: artichokes, asparagus, beet greens, bok choy, broccoli, Brussels sprouts, cabbage, celery, collard greens, kale, lettuce, mustard greens, snap peas, spinach, string beans, Swiss chard, turnip greens, zucchini, herbs (basil, cilantro, dill, oregano, parsley)

Beans: adzuki beans, black beans, black-eyed peas, chickpeas, kidney beans, lentils, lima beans, mung beans, navy beans, pinto beans, soybeans, white beans

Seeds: chia, flax

Rainbow vegetables: avocados, beets, bell peppers, carrots, cauliflower, cucumbers, eggplant, garlic, mushrooms, olives, onions, potatoes, pumpkins, radishes, squash, sweet potatoes, tomatoes, water chestnuts, yams

ARGUMENTS

You could argue that if the goal is to focus on the most nutritious foods, the maximally nutritious diet should consist exclusively of *leafy green vegetables*, which are by far the healthiest edibles on the planet. This is true; however such a diet neglects a few of our criteria. Remember:

For a food to be considered Paradigm, it should be maximally nutritious, innately delicious, available and affordable, properly prepared, environmentally friendly, unrefined, unprocessed and whole.

A bag of mixed greens (collard, mustard, turnip, or spinach), at 100 calories per bag, costs $2.29. A couple of these bags, at under $5, would go far in fulfilling the daily requirements of many major vitamins and minerals. But the average individual needs about 2,000 calories each day to supply energy needs. To satisfy this requirement eating only greens, one would have to consume 20 such bags, at a total cost of nearly $50 per day.

Pricey.

On the other hand, a can of garbanzo beans, while still nutritious - including at least 25 percent of the daily value of 7 essential nutrients - contains over 4 times as many calories (425), while at a mere 89 cents costs less than half as much as our greens. Per calorie, that's one tenth of the price.

An aside: We do not wish to carry the cost per calorie thinking too far. Many consumers have used the *cheap* excuse to justify eating fast food. Example: A 10-piece McDonald's Chicken McNugget Value Meal (with medium fries and medium Coke) provides 1,050 calories, at a total cost of $5, or 200 calories per dollar. That may seem like a deal, until you consider nutrition. The meal provides 0% vitamin A, 17% vitamin C, 4% calcium, and 14% iron. With 48 grams of fat, it should not be considered a steal, unless you're the one getting robbed (of your health, that is). By comparison: For under $3, three cans of kidney beans provides roughly 1,000 calories, 21% vitamin C, 28% calcium and 81% iron – and only 4 grams of fat. Five dollars will buy you 25 bananas: 2,625 calories, 10 grams of fat, 38% vitamin A, 428% vitamin C, 15% calcium, 43% iron and 75 grams of fiber.

Back to our discussion.

A diet exclusively of green vegetables neglects your most important taste bud; the taste bud that detects sweets is on the tip of the tongue and should be satisfied with plenty of sweet fruit. (The other taste buds are salty, sour, bitter and savory, or Umami.)

Additionally, steaming greens, blending them into a shake or tossing them into a salad certainly has ease of preparation on its side, but who in his right mind would deny himself a luscious fruit, which can be eaten right off the tree, whole, unseasoned and raw. A can of beans, rinsed and strained, is ready to eat.

Though leafy greens are the most nutritious of all foods and should feature prominently in your diet, including fruits and beans is a convenient and affordable way to meet calorie needs and supplement nutrition. The colors present in beans and fruits such as apples and berries - red, white, yellow, orange and purple - signal the presence of a vast array of phytonutrients essential to maximal nutrition. And in fact, beans (red, kidney, pinto) and berries comprise 8 of the top 20 antioxidant foods.[53]

Now, you could argue that if we allow fruits and beans, why stop there? Why not include whole grains, nuts and meat? Variety is the spice of life, right? Um, not so much.

BEAT THE MEAT

We've already addressed the differences in the digestive anatomies of humans and carnivores, with human digestion being dependent on fiber and suited to vegetation.

To recap: Meat, eggs and dairy have too much of what we do not require, and not enough of what we do. Animal food supplies an excess amount of protein, which is acidic and growth-promoting and leads to bone disease, kidney and heart problems, obesity and cancer; it is high in fat, much of it in the form of saturated fat and cholesterol, which is rapidly deposited on the hips and the thighs and in the blood vessels; it has not enough vitamins and minerals, little water, no fiber and little or no carbohydrate, our primary energy source, all of which plant food supplies in abundance.

Our innate repugnance to bloodshed, especially if the carcass comes replete with guts, gristle, mucus, feces, teeth, nails and hair, is further proof: Clearly, we were not designed and our diet not meant to include animal protein. In humans, hunting is a learned behavior. No child enthusiastically embraces bloodshed. Animals inspire love and tenderness in us, which is why we keep them as pets. Our pets, on the other hand, are born carnivores. If a cat kept as its pet a parakeet, the bird would quickly wind up as lunch.

But still you wonder, *Where do I get my protein?*

To reiterate, 10 percent of calories from protein, or 50 grams in a 2,000-calorie diet, is more than sufficient to meet the needs of most everyone. Even athletes, bodybuilders and growing kids require no more than this amount.

Mother's milk is often called Mother Nature's perfect food. Indeed it contains all the nutrition necessary to completely sustain the developing infant.[54] Mother's milk is made up of 5 percent protein. Five percent, which Nature in her wisdom deems sufficient to nourish us when we are growing more rapidly than any other point in our lives, effectively doubling our birth weight in 6 months. At puberty, it is common for a 100-lb boy to grow 4 inches and gain 20 pounds in one year. Going from 100 to 120 pounds in 12 months seems like a lot - which is why it is named the *growth spurt* - until you compare this rate of growth (20 percent) to that of the average infant, who grows five times as fast as the adolescent, in half the time, which is like a sixth grader going from 100 to 200 pounds in the same school year. (Sadly, with childhood obesity on the rise, such uncanny weight gain is not uncommon, and it is not associated with a corresponding increase in height. What do grow are the buns, boobs and belly.)

How much protein do infants require in order to achieve this massive growth? Five percent. A diet of strictly lemons and Romaine lettuce would provide 15 percent protein, effectively satisfying the requirement three times over. If eating lettuce dressed in lemon all day seems boring or bland, you may wish simply to emphasize leafy greens and substitute beans wherever you'd normally eat meat. If you are in the habit of having a chicken salad for lunch, try chickpeas instead. Rather than a hamburger patty, mash up a cup of pinto beans. Instead of broiled steak for dinner, boil a blend of beans and greens and you can be sure that your protein need is met.

What's For Dinner?

Protein Comparison: Plant vs. Animal Food

<u>5 oz filet mignon and 1 cup spaghetti</u>
625 calories
33.5 grams protein
34 grams fat
2.5 grams fiber
5 oz water
100% or more DV of vitamin B12, selenium

vs:

<u>1.5 cups lentils and 3 cups boiled spinach</u>
470 calories
43 grams protein
36.5 grams fiber
2.5 grams fat
3 cups water
100% or more DV of 8 nutrients (A, B6, copper, iron, magnesium, manganese, phosphorus, riboflavin)

Meat eaters usually ask vegetarians "Where do you get your protein?" Perhaps it is best to answer this question with a question: "Where do you get your nutrition?" Or, "Where do you get your fiber." The answer to each is the same: "*Not* from meat, bitch." (Profanity not required.) Protein is not lacking in the plant-based diet, but the animal-based diet is devoid of fiber, water and many nutrients.

(Also, notice the reverse relationship of fat and fiber in the plant-based versus the meat-based meals. Plant foods are huge in fiber and low in fat, where the opposite is true with animal foods. But you already knew that!)

There are other health risks associated with eating animal foods. As any microbiologist or gastroenterologist will tell you, gastroenteritis (food poisoning) comes from eating shit, without exception.

And in most cases, the shit comes from the very animals we consume for food.

As digested food, fecal matter is harmless in itself. In fact, roughly 20 percent of your doo doo consists of bacteria, approximately 100,000,000,000 organisms per gram. Yes, that's 1 with 11 zeros after it. One hundred billion bacteria per gram, including a little of the particularly nasty beast that we read about from time to time in the news, E. coli.[55]

And in the intestines, these bacteria serve both a protective and nutritional function. Intestinal bacteria produce vitamins our bodies absorb. And by living on the walls of the colon, the healthy bacteria inhibit the spread of pathogenic (disease-forming) critters that make their way into your insides from time to time. But the bacteria in the colon spell disaster in other parts of the body such as the liver, kidneys, spleen and lungs, which are usually sterile (contain no bacteria). In these and other locations, they are *bacteria non grata* and can cause a *shitload* of damage (pardon the pun).

How do the bacteria in an animal's or another human's insides wind up in your mouth? Obviously, by way of food. The first culprit is the food these animals eat. As an example, let's take cows. The traditional diet of cows consists of grass. In an effort to increase growth rates and produce more meat, many factory farms have taken to feeding cows grains, which as we have seen are more concentrated than plant foods and therefore cause rapid weight gain. However, grains are not the preferred food of cows. (Just as meat is not the preferred food of humans but is meant instead for cats and dogs.) Grains acidify the cow's stomach and encourage the development of acid-resistant bacteria, which replicate in a lower pH and fill the cow's gut. Antibiotics routinely added to the cow's feed to promote growth also contribute to the spread of resistant bacteria. These bacteria can then survive our stomachs, whose acidity is otherwise able to inhibit the growth of organisms and prevent them from going any farther down our pipes.

Okay, I get it, we hear you saying, *factory farming leads to the development of resistant bacteria. But how do the bacteria in cow poop make it to my stomach in the first place?*

When the knife severs the cow's jugular and slices through its belly, it's certainly a bloody mess, and quite deadly if you're the cow. But if the knife happens to slip and slits open the guts, causing fecal matter to spill out, it's a shitty mess, and deadly for humans. It's the ultimate revenge of the harmless creature, who with its watery eyes and a mournful moo, says: *Kill me for food, and then eat my shit.*

It's not just cows that are the source of disease-producing bacteria. Other animals do it too. All the other animals that we consume as food.

The leading cause of food-borne illness in the United States is Campylobacter, primarily from eating **chicken**.

Millions are sickened from eating Salmonella-tainted **eggs** every year.

And the primary source of E. coli infection derives from **cow** manure mixed in with ground beef. Most cases of food poisoning will make you miserable for a couple days and possibly soil your underwear. Not the case with E. coli. Some strains can cause multiple organ failure and death, and if they don't kill you, may leave you blind and epileptic.

Food-borne staphylococcus infections cause nausea and vomiting within hours. The source is usually **dairy products**, for example the potato salad or mayonnaise left in the hot sun at a picnic. Flies are usually to blame in this case, bringing the bacteria in the feces on the ground to the food on the table and making those creams and cheeses so many Petri dishes. Bacteria love warm animal protein. It's the perfect breeding ground, and so they feast on animal foods and reproduce. This is what bacteria do. They are the trash collectors of microorganisms. They clean up the waste, and animal foods, even before they hit the intestines, are waste.

What about the tainted sprouts in Europe, or the spinach or strawberries that sent several to the hospital? The rare cases of food poisoning associated with spinach and other vegetation are invariably due to manure runoff from feedlots, or to poor hygiene in food preparation. It didn't come from the vegetation itself, which actually does a fine job of filtering impurities through its roots and leaves, as we discussed. The source is still the same. In other words, even if you do not eat animal foods, their shit can still smear your food.

It would seem, then, that the best way to eliminate food poisoning is to eliminate animal foods altogether, wash fruits and vegetables prior to consuming and to prepare your own meals.

Pesticides and fertilizer residues are much more concentrated in animal flesh and in milk than they are in produce. In fact, levels of some of the deadliest pesticides are 10 times higher in meat, fish and poultry and 5 times higher in dairy than they are in fruit. And fish is even worse. No fish is free of pollution, and fish including salmon, lobster and sardines, all of which concentrate pollutants in their fat, have 100-times more waste products than the polluted water in which they are bred. Eating sushi is like drinking from an unflushed toilet. And all fish contains mercury, which can cause memory impairment, mental disorders and heart disease. In fact, pregnant women are advised to avoid eating certain types of fish, including swordfish, as toxic levels of mercury may harm the developing fetus. Nursing women, women who are attempting to become pregnant and children as well are advised to do the same and forgo fish.[56] Perhaps this advisory should extend to the rest of the population as well.

In the case of dairy, it should be noted that no animal drinks the milk of another species, or drinks it into adulthood, *except humans*. Humans eat copious amounts of dairy products only to suffer human-specific diseases. Are the two related? Yes. Cow's milk is indigestible by most of us and causes cancer (breast, prostate) and osteoporosis. It is also linked with obesity, diabetes, arthritis, asthma, allergies and ear infections, among many other ailments and afflictions that do not occur in animals. Animals consume the milk of their own species, in infancy and not beyond, and in this respect they should be viewed as the teachers of humanity – that is, if the goal is to be disease-free.

If this is not sufficient argument against dairy consumption, be aware that cow's milk contains morphine derivatives that make it chemically addictive and very difficult to eliminate from the diet. In addition, cow's milk has three times as much protein as mother's milk and contains growth factors including estrogen that increase the risk of cancer and obesity.

Imagine spotting a cow on the side of the road. It is grazing there peacefully and you walk over, stoop down and start sucking on its milk-engorged udders. If that image seems ridiculous to you, how can you reach for the glass of milk or piece of cheese or cup of yogurt and call it natural? The healthy bacteria (probiotics) present in yogurt are unnecessary if you eat a diet full of fibrous fruits and veggies, which feed the healthy bacteria in your gut (you have billions upon billions, remember?) and encourage them to replicate.

Moreover, taken together, fish, eggs and dairy account for more food allergies than any other food. Can a food group that is allergic to so many be healthful for any? In the case of these toxic foods, there is no such thing as moderation.

No is the way to go.

And on to the environmental effects of eating animal foods. Our appetite for flesh is waging a war on Mother Nature, and the loser is the Next Generation, which will inherit the world, and which may include YOU. What kind of world will it be? Depletion of the ozone layer and global warming, manure runoff and water pollution, deforestation and fossil fuel depletion are all occurring at a record-breaking pace. All are courtesy of meat consumption.

All this is fine and well and each taken alone seems convincing enough argument against consuming animal products. But we have neglected to mention the most important reason: to avoid the pain and suffering you participate in, whether you accept it or not, each time an animal is slaughtered or mistreated to please your palate.

Let us assume for a moment that meat is the most nutritious food on the planet, and that humans were designed to eat exclusively animal flesh.

Would this justify inflicting pain on another being and violently ending its life? Are animals not sentient beings like ourselves? Do they not feel pain, scream, shed blood and have nerve endings that are in some cases more sensitive than even our own? (The pig, for example, is very sensitive.) Yes. Should we therefore terrorize them? No, not even if they were the most nutritious food. But as we've shown, animal food is not only nutritiously inferior to plants, it is directly associated with all variety of disease, and cooking meat, by denaturing proteins and deranging fats, makes it more deadly still.

Even in its most pristine form - free-range, grass-fed, organic, raw or lightly cooked - meat is still filthy. As a group, animal products (meat, eggs, dairy) are a haven for unfriendly bacteria, a concentrated source of fat and cholesterol, filled with hormones, antibiotics, heavy metals and toxic chemicals, lacking water and devoid of fiber or energy, making even minimal inclusion in the diet excessive.

Again, no is the way to go.

Organic meat is purportedly raised without the use of drugs, hormones or synthetic chemicals including pesticides and fertilizers. Animals raised on organic farms are supposed to be treated more humanely. However, many animal products labeled *organic* are in fact anything but. There are loopholes in the organic regulations that allow factory farms (which comprise the vast majority of organic producers) to slip their less-than-organic animal products, especially eggs, into the market. These products are less nutritious and the animals are confined and subjected to woeful abuse. Yet, even raising an animal in princely conditions does not excuse condemning it to a violent and premature death. To borrow from Shakespeare: *All's bad that ends bad.*

In short, we cause painful deaths to eat meat, and then by eating meat we in turn suffer painful deaths in the form of cancer, heart disease, kidney failure and strokes. Why not stop the cycle?

The power is yours.

At your next meal, leave the meat and eat your beans and greens. Each time you do, you'll have made the world a better place.

THE CASE AGAINST GRAINS

Grains such as wheat (bread, pasta), oats, barley, rye, rice and quinoa (commonly called a grain but actually a seed) are available and affordable, and whole grains can be modestly nutritious. Refined grains, as in baked goods, most breads, cereals, pastas, bagels, buns and tortillas, are nutritionally bereft. The fiber has been extracted, along with most of the vitamins and minerals. Instead of eating a piece of bread, you may as well devour handfuls of white sugar. Seriously.

Availability, affordability and modest nutrition make whole grains a satisfactory part of a semi-healthy diet, or alternatives to animal foods, but grains are by no means a perfect food. Beans, which are also available and affordable, are nutritionally far superior to grains. And beans come ready-made.

We know what you are thinking: *Beans, beans, good for your heart, the more you eat the more you fart*, and so on. Yes, we've heard this one too. And yes, people often blame their digestive difficulties on the high fiber content of beans. This is simply not the case. As we've shown, many fruits and vegetables including leafy greens and berries have more fiber than even the most fibrous of legumes. In fact, raspberries have over twice as much fiber as pinto beans, yet no one says fruit makes you fart. In truth, fiber facilitates digestion. Foods lacking water and fiber, such as meat and cheese, pose the real threat to gut function. They sit in your intestines for days, fodder for colonic bacteria to ferment, and you know what those little critters produce? Methane (just like cows) and hydrogen gas. That's right, gas. And while the gas at the pumps may smell good to some people, the gas from your gut stinks. You may think it smells like roses, but we beg to differ!

While it is true that GI distress can result from taking in large amounts of fiber at a sitting, for example from bran cereal - which can have as much as 30 grams of fiber per cup, and no water - you are not likely to consume too many beans (15 grams of fiber per cup) to trouble your tract, especially if you eat beans with vegetables, as sprinkled over a salad. If you are new to beans and start by devouring huge bowls at a sitting, then yes you may experience initial stomach discomfort and bloat. However, this quickly subsides as your system accustoms itself to greater intakes of bulk.

In reality, gastrointestinal trouble associated with eating beans is due in most cases to poor food combination. Concentrated (high calorie) foods including rice, tortillas, meat and cheese tax the gut on their own, all the more so if added to the oligosaccharides (starch) present in beans. Soaking beans for one to two days before cooking removes much of these starches and vastly improves digestion, as does eating them with raw or lightly cooked vegetables. Canned beans, so-called poor man's food, are rich in nutrition, inexpensive and convenient. They are packaged in water, so the soaking is done for you. Be sure to select brands with no ingredients other than water (with or without salt), and rinse and strain them well before enjoying. This helps remove the starch residues, and also improves the taste. Start with half a cup of beans per day, and throw out the grains. We mean all that rice and flour, all that bread and barley, those biscuits, buns, bagels and muffins. Be gone, quinoa! Grains simply fail to make the grade.

Tale of the Taste

<u>1 can of black beans (1.5 cups)</u>
340 calories
23 grams protein
22.5 grams of fiber
25% or more of the daily value of 6 nutrients

vs.

<u>1.5 cups cooked brown rice</u>
320 calories
7.5 grams protein
5.2 grams of fiber
25% or more of 3 nutrients

Notice the difference. Beans have 3 times the protein in brown rice and over 4 times the fiber, in addition to twice as many nutrients.

Even quinoa (pronounced keen-WA), highly touted in the health food industry and regarded as a dietary staple by much of the vegan community, does not match up to the protein, fiber or nutritional density of the humble bean, which has twice the fiber and twice the protein.

<u>1.6 cups (300 grams) quinoa</u>
360 calories
12 grams protein
9 grams fiber
25% or more of 5 nutrients

The ratio of unhealthy (omega-6) to healthy (omega-3) fats in brown rice is 22:1. In quinoa the ratio is 11:1. The polyunsaturated fat ratio in beans? Roughly 1:1.

Inferior nutrition aside, there are other problems with grains. And it only begins with the fact that grains, in their raw, natural state, are totally unappealing to the senses. Imagine that you were starving and came upon a field of wheat. Would your first impulse be to pounce on those dry, brittle stalks and eat your fill? Only if you were crazy. Now replace that wheat field with an orange grove, or a strawberry patch, or a row of sun-drenched apple trees bursting with fruit. How does sinking your teeth into a juicy fruit and eating your heart's content sound? You'd have to be crazy to pass it up!

No conversation about wheat would be complete without mentioning one of its major components. You may have heard of gluten. Gluten is the protein found in wheat. It is also found in barley and rye, and it is a potent food allergen. In fact, it causes celiac disease, also known as wheat sensitivity. To get scientific for a moment, celiac sprue, as it is also called, is a malabsorptive state characterized by inflammation of the small intestine with or without itchy skin eruptions (dermatitis herpetiformis). That's what the medical textbooks will tell you. Basically, your body develops an immune response to gluten and goes on attack. The sensitive cells of the small intestine are damaged and consequently can no longer perform their function, which is to absorb nutrients. So you are left with the symptoms of sprue, which as with lactose intolerance include gas, bloat, abdominal pain and diarrhea.

More than 2 million Americans have been diagnosed with celiac disease, which runs in families. Many more have the condition but are unaware. This may include you. According to the National Institutes of Health, one person might have diarrhea and abdominal pain, while another person may be irritable or depressed. Irritability is one of the most common symptoms in children.[57] Irritability? Depression? What do irritability and depression have to do with poor digestion? A lot, it seems. Remember, you are only as healthy as your gut. If you have ever been irritable, you know that it can make it difficult to concentrate. Irritability can in fact decrease attention span, which can lead to a diagnosis of ADHD, or Attention deficit/hyperactivity disorder, and its sequelae: poor grades and angry outbursts. So you or your child gets put on amphetamines, which are the treatment of choice for ADHD. Amphetamines can lead to stunted growth in kids, in addition to digestive difficulties, as if your life wasn't already hard enough! The failure to properly absorb nutrients can also stunt growth. In short, who wants to be short?

Finally, because grains are higher in sugar and lower in fiber relative to plant foods, grains have higher **glycemic values**. Another five dollar phrase.

Glycemic Index

The glycemic index measures the effect different carbohydrates have on blood sugar levels. A body in perfect working order can handle large amounts of ingested carbohydrate, no problem. As we have seen, carbs are quickly broken down into the simple sugars, glucose and fructose, and then absorbed. (Again, the exception is the disaccharide lactose. By the age of 3, many humans no longer produce the enzyme lactase, which breaks down lactose. The result is lactose intolerance. It seems from this that we were not meant to ingest milk much after infancy.)

As mentioned, both fructose and glucose are present in most carbohydrate foods, as starch, as pairs (sucrose), or in their free form.

Fructose, the sweetest of all sugars, is found in fruits and vegetables. Glucose is also present in fruit, but it exists in higher concentrations in processed foods with added sugar. You know: colas, candies, breads and pastries. Consider that one small (16-oz) Coke has a whopping 47 grams of sugar, whereas one cup of strawberries has barely 7 grams. That's a seven-fold difference!

Insulin is the body's response to ingested glucose. It promotes the entrance of glucose into cells. Called the hormone of plenty, insulin also causes fat synthesis and storage. Its presence signals the body that a surplus of calories is on-hand, so it's okay to save some for the proverbial rainy day. If too much insulin is around, however, the blood glucose level can go from too high to too low too quickly. The result? The symptoms of hunger, dizziness, lightheadedness, weakness, fatigue and food cravings. Low blood sugar convinces your body that you are starving, and so you grab whatever munchies are at hand. As more sugary food goes down your gullet, blood sugar rises, leading to more insulin, which causes the blood sugar to plummet, and the cravings return and the vicious cycle repeats itself. The result: You pack on pounds!

Unlike glucose, fructose does not promote the release of insulin. (Research linking fructose with cancer tends to use the artificial sweetener high-fructose corn syrup, which is pure sugar. The fructose found naturally in fruits, packed in water and fiber, does not support tumor growth. It supports health.)

Most of us begin life with the ability to release just the right amount of insulin for an ingested quantity of glucose. With time and poor food choices, your body loses this sensitivity, your pancreas puts out too much insulin, blood sugar plummets and eventually the pancreas gets burned out. Without enough insulin to drive sugar into the cells that really need it, such as your muscles, you tire easily. To make matters worse, when glucose remains in the blood it damages the vessels, nerves, eyes, kidneys and skin. At its worst, diabetes, which is a disease of insulin deficiency and ineffectiveness, results in blindness, kidney failure and gangrene. Not fun. So you can't find your way to the toilet, but without the use of your kidneys, you won't be needing the toilet anyway, an optimist might say.

Of course this is an extreme scenario, but it serves to illustrate why it is important to eat low glycemic foods, starting, like, yesterday! Such foods discourage blood sugar abnormalities, constant cravings and weight gain, while higher glycemic foods encourage these inconveniences.

So, what exactly is the glycemic index? The **glycemic index** is determined by administering a quantity of food (usually 50 grams of carbohydrate) and measuring its effect on blood sugar over time (usually two hours). As a reference point, pure glucose – the essence of blood sugar – gets a score of 100%, or 100. Since no food is made of pure glucose, pure glucose raises blood sugar more than any food, and so all values are necessarily less than 100. For example, strawberry jam, consisting almost purely of nearly equal parts glucose and fructose, has a glycemic index of 50%, or 50, which means that it has half the effect on blood sugar (and on insulin) that pure glucose has.

The **glycemic load** is the amount of carbohydrate in a serving of food multiplied by its glycemic index. Few foods are pure carbohydrate. Most have at least some protein and fat, and since protein and fat have negligible effects on blood glucose, the glycemic load better reflects a food's impact on one's biochemistry than glycemic index.

To elucidate: Protein and fat (and water and fiber) all decrease the carbohydrate content in a serving of food. The more protein and fat in food, the fewer calories derive from carbohydrate. And since serving sizes are often by weight (grams), water and fiber, which are both non-caloric, add weight and decrease calories, and therefore carbohydrate in a serving of a given food. Confused yet? Then get this: Less carbohydrate means less effect on blood sugar.

Taking the example of strawberry jam, which has 20 grams of carbohydrate per serving. Twenty times 50% (the glycemic index of jam) gives us 10 (20 x .5 = 10; half of 20 is 10). The glycemic load of strawberry jam is therefore 10. By contrast, fresh strawberries have a glycemic load of 1. Yes, 1.

Anything below 55 is considered a low glycemic index food. Anything below 10 has a low glycemic load.

Here are the glycemic values of some common foods:[58]

Food	Glycemic Index	Glycemic Load
spinach	0	0
orange	31	3
apple	38	6
orange juice	46	12
carrots	47	3
kidney beans	**25**	**6**
watermelon	72	4
	---------	
quinoa	53	13
oatmeal	58	13
pasta	42	20
brown rice	68	22
white rice	64	23
bagel	69	24
Grape-Nuts	71	29

As you can see, whether whole or refined, grains have high glycemic values, double and in some cases quintuple (5 times) that of beans, higher even than sweet fruit. Moreover, many vegetables are so low in sugar that they don't even have a glycemic index. Even those that do — take starchy vegetables such as sweet potatoes (44;11)- have lower values than grains. And in the case of sweet potatoes and fruits such as bananas and dates that have higher glycemic values, their high fiber content works to slow the absorption of sugar and prevents energy ups and downs. One medium banana, for example, has 3 grams of fiber, which is double the amount of fiber found in a serving of brown rice.

If you are worried about your blood sugar or have insulin resistance or diabetes that requires you to monitor the sugar content in foods, you do not need to avoid your favorite sweet juicy fruits. The glycemic index evaluates a food on its own, but rarely do we eat one food at a time, and here we can use food combination to our advantage. You see, high glycemic fruits may be combined with lower glycemic foods to reduce the effect on blood sugar. Bananas if eaten alone have a glycemic load of 13, but when consumed with an equal portion of oranges, the value falls to 8. Just be sure to eat whole oranges, rather than merely drink the juice. Without the fiber in the whole food, the sugar in oranges and other fruits can mess with your glucose levels. For the adventurous, blending fruits with leafy greens (which are glycemic-free), or mixing a cup or 2 of baby spinach into your fruit salad, helps to *lower the load* (glycemic load, that is).

What about animal products? It is true that most animal foods (meat and eggs) are so low in carbohydrates as to have no glycemic values. Milk, which contains the sugar lactose, is the lone exception. However, animal foods promote the release of insulin, which is tantamount to being a high glycemic food, without the energy spike that comes with, say, eating a candy bar. In fact, milk (both whole and skimmed) elicits a **disproportionately large insulin response** relative to its low glycemic load of 5.[59] The result is weight gain, fatigue and other symptoms of hyperinsulinemia. Chalk that up as another strike against animal foods.

To review, high glycemic foods - and some low glycemic animal foods - lead to insulin spikes, blood sugar imbalances, overeating, fat storage and disease.

As if inferior nutrition and exorbitant glycemic values wasn't enough to dump the bread, be mindful that as a group, grains are a concentrated food. They have lots of calories per mouthful, and are simply too easy to overeat. Without water and fiber, your body doesn't get the message that it's full until your mouth has gobbled down too many cookies. Remember this the next time you reach for that second muffin.

Additionally, grains are acid-forming, which disrupts your body's pH balance. By contrast, legumes such as lentils, peas, lima beans, white beans, navy beans and soybeans are alkalinizing, as are starchy vegetables including zucchini.

It follows therefore that to fulfill your carb cravings, beans are best, and starchy vegetables will do. In fact, potatoes, pumpkins and squash (and let's not forget bananas) make great substitutes for grain cravings. If you find yourself desiring pasta, try making it out of spaghetti squash or zucchini. If you crave pastries, a sweet potato is just as satisfying, and far more nutritious. Normally have oatmeal with raisins for breakfast? Have a few bananas instead.

In summary, grains are hardly the health foods they seem. Even breads labeled *whole wheat* or *whole grain* can contain large amounts of refined flour and relatively small portions of whole grains. As with most packaged foods, manufacturers have subtle methods at their disposal for disguising deleterious ingredients and making them appear more nutritious than they are.[60] And even products that are 100 percent whole grain contain anti-nutrients that inhibit the functioning of the very digestive enzymes (proteases, amylases) on which their breakdown depends.[61]

The conclusion is irrefutable: If you want tight buns, drop that hamburger bun now!

NUTS, GO!

Many nutritional experts tout the benefits of eating nuts. While these foods may offer protection against certain forms of disease, fruits and vegetables offer more protection, at a fraction of the calories and fat, and with more vitamins, minerals and fiber and far more water. Compare these two snacks:

1 oz almonds (about 25 nuts)
185 calories
18.5 grams fat
2 grams fiber
25% or more of 1 nutrient

vs.

3 cups strawberries
147 calories
1.5 grams fat
9 grams fiber
25% or more of 3 nutrients

As with grains, nuts have more against them than nutritional inferiority. First is the issue of how they are commercially prepared. Nuts usually come roasted and salted. The roasting process exposes them to very high heat (over 400 degrees Fahrenheit, twice the boiling point of water); this causes the depletion of fat-soluble vitamins such as vitamin E, and the formation of free radicals. Remember these? To review, free radicals are highly reactive molecules that cause chain reactions of destruction, aging and death. Many commercially packaged nuts and seeds are cooked in hydrogenated oils, adding the deadly trans fat to the diet. The added salt in nuts can increase blood pressure, contribute to kidney stones and leech the bones of minerals.

Raw, unsalted nuts are a better option. They can be good sources of certain nutrients, including vitamin E and the mineral selenium. However, nuts have an extraordinarily high amount of the pro-inflammatory fatty acid omega-6. One cup of raw peanuts, for example, has over 20,000 mg of omega-6, and only 4.4 mg of omega-3. This is a ratio of over 4,000 to 1!

Also, tree nuts (almonds, walnuts, cashews, etc.) and peanuts are recognized by the USDA as major food allergens. The others are wheat, soybeans, eggs, milk and fish.[62] Corn, which is one of the most common genetically modified foods (GMO), has been implicated in many food sensitivities as well. Other common GMOs are soybeans, canola oil (rapeseed), tomatoes and potatoes. The American Academy of Environmental Medicine notes that health risks associated with GM food consumption include **infertility, immune dysregulation, intestinal damage** and **accelerated aging**, as several animal studies have indicated.[63]

According to the FDA, millions suffer food allergies each year, although many symptoms are so mild as to go undiagnosed. In other words, you may not know that you and your family are allergic to dairy, wheat, soy, eggs, milk, fish or nuts, but if you experience congestion, dry cough, stomach upset, asthma, diarrhea or constipation, swelling of the face or eyes, flatulence or fatigue, you likely are intolerant to one or more of these foods. And who doesn't suffer these symptoms! There is no cure for allergies other than strict avoidance. It is recommended that symptom sufferers eliminate potential allergens from the diet until symptoms disappear, then reintroduce foods one at a time to identify the culprit. This can be time-consuming and confusing. Why not just delete all wheat, soybeans, eggs, milk products, fish and corn from your diet once and for all? This goes for nuts as well.

Those who suffer from herpes simplex outbreaks should take particular care to avoid nuts, which have high levels of the amino acid arginine. Herpes is very common in the general population. By the time you are a teenager or young adult, chances that you have been infected with oral herpes (HSV-1) are 1 in 2, or 50 percent. By age 50, this figure rises to over 80 percent.[64] Type 2, commonly called genital herpes, has a prevalence of over 15 percent, meaning 1 of every 6 people has it.[65]

Herpes simplex causes painful, itchy lesions on the mouth, genitals or buttocks. There is no cure for the herpes virus, which lies dormant in the nerves of your spine only to reactivate in times of stress or immunosuppression. It is not known why some are more susceptible to herpes outbreaks than others, but diet has been shown to be a major influence. In order to replicate, the herpes virus requires arginine, while the amino acid lysine competes with arginine and suppresses outbreaks.[66] In other words, the more arginine in the diet, and the less lysine consumed, the greater the likelihood that a lesion will occur, and the more severe it will be. Without exception, nuts have several times more arginine than lysine. One hundred grams of walnuts, for instance, contains 2,500 mg arginine to 450 mg lysine, a ratio of over 5 to 1. This, coincidentally, is similar to the ratio found in walnuts of omega-6 to omega-3, another reason to say NO to them.

Like nuts, many grains (wheat, oats) are high in arginine and contribute to herpes outbreaks, as does chocolate. By comparison, in nutritional yeast this ratio is reversed. One serving of yeast has nearly twice as much lysine as arginine (918 mg to 510 mg) and may help to suppress herpes outbreaks. Yeast has many other benefits, which we will get to presently.

And the list goes on...

Most nuts are encased in a hard shell. As such, it does not seem that nature intended for nuts to be eaten in large quantities, as people commonly due at sporting events, happy hour or sitting in front of the TV mindlessly shoveling handfuls down the throat. Historically, our ancestors struggled with their bare hands and rudimentary tools to crack open the shells of even a few nuts - and by doing so they probably burned many calories, if only in sheer frustration! But shelled and in bulk, nuts lend themselves to overindulgence. A serving of nuts is 1 oz, which is about 20 nuts, or one palm-sized portion. One can easily devour several of these 200-calorie handfuls at a sitting, totaling a thousand or more calories. (This is our personal confession. Guilty as charged!) Nut butters are even more concentrated. A heaping spoonful of peanut butter can exceed 400 calories, which is more than an entire can of lentils.

<u>1 heaping helping of peanut butter (4 rounded tbsp)</u>
375 calories
32.5 grams of fat
under 4 grams fiber
0% vitamin C, 3% calcium, 7% iron

vs.

<u>1 can of lentils</u>
340 calories
1.1 grams fat

23.5 grams fiber
7% vitamin C, 6% calcium, 55% iron

Note that the fat-to-fiber ratio of lentils is the opposite of the ratio in nuts: Lentils have over 20 times more fiber than fat, while peanut butter has roughly 10 times more fat than fiber.

Not only are nuts and nut butters a concentrated source of calories and fat, they are oftentimes poorly combined (with jellies, jams and dried fruit) or eaten with other concentrated foods, as on bread or with pretzels. This significantly increases the calorie load and is of further burden to the digestion. And we haven't even discussed how dry nuts are. They contain no water at all, which dries your mouth, clogs your throat, upsets your stomach and shrinks your cells. Their lack of water content is probably why nuts are so often consumed with beer. Sadly, beer's diuretic effect compounds the cell-shrinking quality of nuts and makes a desert wasteland of your blood vessels and tissues!

Furthermore (we're almost done) nuts as well as many seeds are overt fats, meaning they derive the bulk of their calories (70 percent or more) from fat. Macadamia nuts are nearly 90 percent fat. And as mentioned this fat is mainly in the pro-inflammatory omega-6 form, which produces free radicals that contribute to premature aging, cancer and chronic diseases.

FOCUS ON FAT

1 oz sunflower seeds (163 calories)
13.5 grams total fat
1.5 grams saturated fat
2.8 grams monounsaturated fat
9.2 grams polyunsaturated fat
9.180 grams omega-6
0.020 grams omega-3

As noted, even without overt fat in the diet, fruits and vegetables alone easily meet your requirement of 10 percent of calories from dietary fat. If you desire or require additional dietary fat, the ideal sources are the fatty fruits, olives and avocados, which contain high amounts of monounsaturated fatty acids, more water and more fiber than their nutty counterparts.

OVERT FATS COMPARED

½ avocado
140 calories
13 grams fat (mostly monounsaturated)
6 grams of fiber
2 oz water

or:

30 large black olives
150 calories
14 grams of fat (mostly monounsaturated)
4 grams fiber
4 oz water
11% DV vitamin A, 2% vitamin C, 12% calcium, 24% iron.

VS.

1 oz almonds (about 25)
165 calories
14.5 grams fat (mostly polyunsaturated)
3.5 grams fiber
0 water
0% DV vitamin A, 0% vitamin C, 7% calcium, 7% iron.

or:

1 tbsp olive oil
180 calories
20 grams of fat
0 grams of fiber
0 water
no nutrients

From this, it would seem that the best option is to avoid nuts and oils altogether. An occasional handful of nuts may be okay, but as we've shown it is unrealistic to consider them health foods, because in excessive amounts they can do more harm than help. Still, nuts are better than pork loin, so you're headed in the right direction.

In the case of seeds, since our genetic cousins the chimpanzees eat them, maybe so should we, but a little goes a long way. If you include seeds in your dietary regimen, opt for flax or chia seeds, which are unprocessed, unsalted and not likely to be overindulged in; moreover, flax and chia are the only seeds that contain a large amount of omega-3 fats. Be sure to grind the flax seed just prior to using. They are good blended in a smoothie or sprinkled over a salad. Or, you might try sprouting sunflower seeds. Sprouting lowers the fat content and increases the nutritional value. Both bean (soy, mung, garbanzo, lentil) and seed sprouts make delicious additions to a salad.

To sprout, buy a Mason jar (32-oz) with a perforated lid. Fill with water. Add ½ cup dried, raw, organic beans or seeds, cover and soak for 24 hours. Drain the water. Rinse and strain the beans/seeds once daily for 3 to 5 days. Keep out of direct sunlight. Once the sprouts fill the jar, they are ready to eat. Leftovers may be stored uncovered in the refrigerator for up to one week.

* * *

Now that we are convinced that the maximally nutritious foods are plants and plants alone, we can determine whether these plant foods meet our other criteria and deserve the term *Paradigm*.

COURSE TWO: THE OTHER CRITERIA

For a food to be considered Paradigm, it should be maximally nutritious, innately delicious, available and affordable, properly prepared, environmentally friendly, unrefined, unprocessed and whole.

INNATELY DELICIOUS

Innate deliciousness is the quality of a food in its natural, unprocessed state to appeal to our sense of taste.

Are plants delicious? Do they cause us to salivate when we are hungry and behold them in their natural state? Consider the apple. Sweet, juicy, refreshing. Or the cucumber. Crisp, crunchy and invigorating. The fig is smooth and succulent. The banana is hearty and fulfilling. Sprouted beans, with their hint of spice, are mouthwatering, lip-smacking and satisfying. In fact, no food other than plants is appealing naturally but how we make it so through cooking and by the addition of various chemicals (oils, colorings, flavorings) and seasonings.

Now, you may be saying that you do not naturally gravitate to certain vegetables. It is true that raw and unseasoned asparagus or Brussels sprouts is not all that appealing unless you are quite hungry, if not downright starving. Moreover, certain members of the legume family contain anti-nutrients that interfere with digestion unless neutralized in the cooking process, and most beans do not appeal to our appetites in their raw state. They're like little tasteless pebbles!

How do we resolve this apparent inconsistency between the diet we recommend and the foods we choose to consume uncooked? If you are a purist and wish to eat only those foods that appeal to you in their raw state, by all means do so. Go with your senses. Let them lead. Eat only the natural foods your taste buds gravitate to. A diet of fresh fruit, vegetable fruits (cucumbers, tomatoes, avocado, bell peppers, olives) and perhaps a few other vegetables, such as celery, carrots, snap peas and mushrooms, with some added leafy greens and herbs (spinach, basil, lettuce) and perhaps some seeds (flax, chia) would delight even the finickiest of eaters. And its sublime nutritiousness has sustained many a raw foodist. But such a diet would deprive you of a large group of vegetables that if lightly cooked and seasoned are utterly irresistible. And yes, this includes asparagus, beans and Brussels sprouts.

In contrast to even the fibrous vegetable, most meats would cause you to vomit if you ate them raw. Manufacturers know this and so they process meat, usually beyond recognition, plucking the hair, removing the claws, feet and intestines and washing away the blood before subjecting the wretched creatures some call *food* to high temperatures while adding copious amounts of salt and fat. Even raw foods such as sushi/sashimi are not in their natural state. The fish is skinned, deboned, cleansed of blood, soaked in wasabe and soy sauce - and often washed down with sake. You almost have to be drunk to enjoy those slimy suckers. Taking a bite out of a fish as it appears in nature, or dangling from the hook, would induce the gag reflex, certainly. The smell alone is repulsive!

Wait a minute, you're saying, *you may be right about old dirty meat smelling disgusting, but who doesn't salivate at the sight of a greasy hamburger!*

You are right. You do. We all do. But just because you salivate over cooked flesh doesn't mean you should eat it. Processed food is designed to seduce our taste buds, and the added fat, salt and sugar play on primordial urges that governed our evolution over the course of millions of years. We are designed to seek out fat (read: French fries, greasy burgers, bags of peanuts) and devour it until we are fed to the teeth. Remember, famine was the prevailing condition for most of human evolution. He who could eat the most fat could survive the longest during famine. But now that we live in a time of plenty, our evolutionary urges no longer serve us. In fact, they do us a disservice and only serve to make us fat. So yes, you will always crave meat and salivate at the smell of fried fat, but this doesn't mean these foods are meant for you. Even crack addicts know that the drugs they hanker after are no good for them. The point is to exercise willpower and stay away from the temptation of intoxicating foods, by surrounding yourself with foods that are nutritious and delicious.

Plant foods are not only nutritious and delicious; they are also satisfying. Feeling satisfaction from food involves a complex interplay of factors, from stretch receptors in our stomach to nutrient receptors in the intestines. Satisfaction differs from satiation, or feeling full to excess, which is an indication merely that you ate sufficient (or often excessive) quantities of food. In fact, foods that satisfy actually *prevent* satiation.

To feel satisfied, you need to eat enough bulk. In fact, the average American consumes 5.5 lbs of food each day.[67] You also need to consume enough nutrients, and over a long enough period of time, as the body doesn't register fullness until at least 20 minutes following the first bite.

If either the need for bulk or the need for nutrition is not met, the tendency is to overeat, either by stuffing oneself, or by snacking indiscriminately and continuously. If you meet these needs with food that lacks the bulk provided by water and fiber, you will consume too many calories and put on pounds. Here is the caloric content in 5 lbs of several common foods.

5 LBS' WORTH
spinach: 520 calories
peaches: 885 calories
carrots: 930 calories
red potatoes: 1,585 calories
kidney beans: 1,925 calories
pasta: 2,950 calories
salmon: 3,150 calories
cheese: 9,150 calories
cashews: 13,177 calories
olive oil: 20,050 calories

You see, foods with water and fiber are naturally low in calories, so you don't have to restrict yourself to small portions. Why eat like a teenage girl on her first date when you can enjoy lbs of fresh fruits and vegetables, guilt-free? Though filling and called *heavy* by some, beans are much lower in calories than grains, meats, nuts, dairy and oils. In fact, 5 lbs of kidney beans nicely coincides with your daily caloric needs, providing nearly 2,000 calories. While satisfying your need for bulk, beans supply nearly 150 grams of fiber, 120 grams of protein, and over 100 percent of the daily requirement for 8 major nutrients. However, if you opted to devote the day to eating cheese instead, by satisfying your bulk requirements and eating 5 lbs of Parmesan you would have consumed 7,000 calories too many, which equals 2 lbs of belly flab.

Lesson to be learned: As the water and fiber content in your food diminishes, calories increase, body weight balloons and fat storage skyrockets.

The only way to feel truly satisfied is to choose foods that are nutritious, bulky (high in water and fiber) and require thorough chewing, which lets them hit all your taste receptors and allows for the sensation of satisfaction to sink in. Once again, the prescription is plants, which have the added benefit of being naturally delicious.

This is not to say that spices and seasonings cannot be used to complement flavor. They can and should be. It is preferable that condiments contain as few (5 or less) ingredients as possible. The following suggestions have ingredients which are both few in number and all-natural:

Dijon mustard: piquant; brings life to even the simplest dish. (Ingredients: mustard seed, salt, vinegar, citric acid, wine.)
Bragg's Liquid Aminos: This soy sauce alternative is made with organic soybeans, contains only a fraction of the sodium and none of the wheat. (Ingredients: Vegetable protein from soybeans and purified water.)
Olive tapenade: all of the nutrition present in the whole olive, and only one-third of the fat and calories of olive oil. (Ingredients: Olives, capers, garlic, lemon, and pepper.) *Be sure to buy the brands with no added oil!*
Tabasco sauce: 3 ingredients – vinegar, peppers and salt – really spice things up.
Lemons: The juice of one lemon mixed with some garlic, mustard, and hot sauce is the perfect salad dressing; no oil or vinegar needed.
Nutritional yeast: This nutritional powerhouse lends a nutty, cheesy flavor to salads and sautés.

Coconut milk: Available in a can, coconut milk adds a creaminess to select dishes. Coconuts are high in saturated fat, so choose *light* varieties. The added water greatly reduces fat content. A can of *light* coconut milk has as many calories and as much fat as a can of olives (250 calories) so use sparingly. Try mixing with nutritional yeast for added savor.

Miscellaneous seasoning (to impart an ethnic flavor): cayenne, turmeric, chili flakes, pepper, cumin, etc.

Salt: Instead of salt, use potassium salt (Lo-salt or No-salt; Morton's brand makes comparable products). Potassium salt tastes like regular salt but has little or no sodium, so it won't increase your blood pressure or cause other health problems including stomach cancer and osteoporosis, which may be linked to excessive dietary sodium. Of course, as we've said athletes have higher sodium requirements than sedentary folk due to the losses that occur in sweat, so if you are active you may prefer to enjoy regular salt with your evening meal.

AVAILABLE AND AFFORDABLE

In contrast to premium foods and supplements, which are usually only found at health food and vitamin stores, an available food can be purchased at the local market. Fruits and vegetables are available year round in most stores, if not fresh then frozen, which is just as good. Yes, some nutrients are damaged in the freezing process. But frozen fruits are picked and packaged at the peak of ripeness. This is an added plus. (So many P's!)

Affordability is trickier. Budgets vary by family. Even so-called "Value Meals" differ in price depending on the city, from under $4.00 to over $8.00. Let us go with an average cost of a fast-food meal of $5.00. Three such meals a day brings us to $15.00, or $105.00 for the week, per person. This is considered affordable by the standards of most.

(Fast food is often considered a source of cheap calories. It is important to remember, however, that in terms of nutrition, a fast-food meal is actually quite pricey. If instead of cost per calorie we considered cost per nutrient, one would have to eat many burgers and fries to approach the nutrition in a single leaf of spinach, and likely never get there.)

So, with $105 spending cash, are we able to purchase enough produce to meet our weekly caloric and nutritional requirements? A recent trip to our local store produced these findings:

One bag of mixed leafy greens (4 servings): $2.29.
One can of beans: 89 cents.
One lb of dates (1,200 calories): $3.69.
Bananas: 19 cents each.
Four lbs of peaches (12 peaches, or 3 per pound): $4.99.

This is about 40 cents per peach. Let's say you chose to eat all 12 peaches for lunch (there are those who do). Would your nutritional requirements be satisfied?

<u>12 peaches: $4.99</u>
calories: 450
carbohydrate: 110 grams
protein: 11 grams
fat: 3 grams
fiber: 17.5 grams
ratio: 87-8-5
Includes 25% or more DV of 12 essential nutrients.

In addition, such a lunch would provide over 4 cups of water (1.05 L), so you won't need to visit the fountain or buy an Evian. Overall, not bad. Compare this with:

<u>A Big Mac Meal (burger, medium fries, medium Coke): $5.79</u>
calories: 1,130
carbohydrate: 151 grams
protein: 29 grams
fat: 48 grams
fiber: 8 grams
ratio: 52-10-38
Includes 25% or more DV of 2 essential nutrients.

The two meals provide roughly the same percentage of calories from protein (8 to 10 percent). For almost a dollar more, the "Value Meal" gets you twice as many calories, but it also gets you 6 times the fat, less than half the amount of fiber and only one tenth of the nutritional value, measured as an average percent per nutrient of all major vitamins and minerals.

Getting back to our point, let us see whether we can purchase a week's worth of groceries (fruits, vegetables, beans and condiments) for $105. But first, to know what is considered a week's worth of groceries, we must identify our target food intake.

DAILY FOOD INTAKE

1. One lb of raw vegetables and vegetable fruits (100 calories).

This is equivalent to 1 head of Romaine lettuce or 3 large red peppers, either of which delivers 100 calories. Other examples include 4 large carrots, 3 large tomatoes or 3 large cucumbers.

These examples are provided as a reference. It is not to say that you must consume a pound of a particular vegetable, though you certainly could. Many prefer mixing various vegetables together in a salad or eating a platter of assorted sliced vegetables before lunch or dinner.

2. One lb of cooked vegetables (100 cals).

This equals 3 cups boiled spinach or 3 cups cooked broccoli, also 100 calories.

Together, one lb of cooked vegetables and one lb of raw vegetables provides the bulk of the day's *nutrients*, at only a fraction (200, or 10 percent) of the day's *calories*. Eating them is like taking a multivitamin with added nutrients and the additional benefits of water and fiber.

For example, one lb of Romaine lettuce, plus one lb of steamed broccoli (70-19-11), provides 230 calories, 21 grams of fiber, and 50 percent or more of the DV for 10 essential vitamins and minerals, including vitamins A, B1, B2, B5, B6 and C; iron, manganese, phosphorus and potassium.

3. One or 2 cans/cups of beans (350 to 700 cals), and/or 1 or 2 starchy vegetables

Beans are a ready-made, nutritious, inexpensive, relatively concentrated source of calories, protein and fiber.

Two cans of beans (one kidney, one garbanzo) provides 750 calories, 38 grams protein, 40 grams fiber and 50 percent or higher of 7 essential nutrients.

Starchy vegetables (potatoes, sweet potatoes, squash) provide concentrated calories that are very satisfying.

4. Two or 3 servings (150 calories each) of fatty fruit.

Olives and avocados provide a healthy dose of healthy fat, and add a savory quality to vegetable dishes.

Example:

One half an avocado and 15 large olives (soaked in water) supplies approximately 250 calories and 20 grams of mainly monounsaturated fat.

Additionally or alternatively, you may wish to include 1 or 2 tbsp of either flax or chia seeds, for the benefit of extra omega-3.

5. Three to 4 lbs of sweet fruit (8 to 12 standard servings, which total roughly 800 calories).

High in water and fiber, fruit provides additional bulk to the diet and is a worthy source of calories, vitamins and some minerals. It also satisfies the sweet tooth.

Example:

One lb of bananas (4 medium), one lb of oranges (4 medium) and one lb of raspberries (4 cups) provides 850 calories, 50 grams fiber and greater than 50 percent of the DV for 12 nutrients.

Taken together, here's how the above foods add up:

Calories: 2,100
Ratio: 75-11-14
Fiber: 123 grams
That's perfection!

IN SUMMARY

Each day we should aim to consume:

**One lb of raw vegetables and vegetable fruit,
One lb of cooked vegetables,
Two to 4 servings of beans/potatoes
Two or 3 servings of fatty fruit,
Three or 4 lbs of sweet fruit.**

These staples fit nicely into a diet as follows:

**Breakfast: fruit shake
Mid-morning snack: fruit salad or individual fruits
Lunch: large salad and/or more fruit
Dinner: raw vegetables and one or two lightly cooked vegeta-
bles, with or without beans/potatoes
Dessert: fresh fruit, if desired.**

Can we purchase enough of these foods (fruits, vegetables, beans) to prepare such a menu for a week, at $105 or less? Here is a recent grocery bill from our local Trader Joe's market:

Fruits
(22 lbs)
4 peaches: $1.99
1 lb figs: $1.99
1 mini watermelon: $2.99
1 lb organic green grapes: $2.99
1 lb organic kiwis: $2.29
2 lb medjool dates: $7.38
28 bananas: $5.38
2 cantaloupes: $1.98
1 honeydew melon: $2.99
3 bags (12 oz each) frozen berries: $8.97

Vegetable fruits
3 large avocados: $3.87
5 tomatoes: $1.99
4 organic cucumbers: $4.98

6-pack bell peppers: $6.98
1 can pitted extra-large olives: $1.49

Vegetables
1 can artichoke hearts in water: $1.99
red and green leaf lettuce: $1.99
3 bags wild arugula: $5.97
2 bags steaming greens: $4.58
2 onions: $1.18
3 bunches peeled garlic: $1.99
1 lb Brussels sprouts: $1.99
1 bag frozen stir fry vegetables: $2.29
1 bag broccoli: $1.99
1 cauliflower: $1.79
1 box (12 oz) crimini mushrooms: $2.99

Beans
1 lb frozen ready to eat edamame: $1.69
6 cans of beans (kidney, garbanzo, pinto): $5.34

Condiments
hot sauce: $1.99
olive tapenade: $3.49
Dijon mustard: $1.69
1 lb organic lemons: $1.99

Total: $103.20

As you can see, we are able to buy a superabundance of produce for the week - three meals plus dessert - for less than what it would cost to eat three daily meals at McDonald's. Here's how we might apply this food to a day's menu.

SAMPLE MENU

Breakfast: Fruit shake

A fruit shake is an excellent way to start the day. In fact, there really is no better way. Blending fruit assures it is thoroughly broken down for rapid absorption and instant energy. In fact, liquid meals leave the stomach twice as rapidly as solid ones.[68]

The ideal shake needs no juice or liquid of any kind, not even water. Three ingredients suffice:

1. **juicy fruit** (melons, citrus) provides the liquid; water is another option
2. **concentrated fruit** (bananas, dates) provides the sweetness and the calories; chia or flax is another option
3. **high ORAC fruits** (the top scoring antioxidant fruits include blueberries, blackberries, strawberries and raspberries) provide the antioxidant kick

You may add a fourth ingredient if you have this shake for lunch and are really hard core:

4. **a leafy green** (spinach) provides additional phytonutrients

Cost
2 cups watermelon: $1.50
2 frozen bananas: 38 cents
½ bag of frozen blueberries: $1.49
1 serving of mixed greens (optional): 57 cents

Directions: Add the melon first and blend to liquid. Then add the frozen berries, bananas and mixed greens. If additional calories are desired, add any combination of bananas, dates, prunes, or even avocado (rich and creamy: give it a try!). Sweeten with cocoa powder, cinnamon and/or stevia.

Mid-morning snack: Fruit salad
2 peaches: 98 cents
1 banana: 38 cents

Lunch: Greens and beans
1 bag (3 cups) broccoli: $1.99
1 can of beans: 89 cents
2 tomatoes: 80 cents

Dinner: Salad and steamed vegetables
1 lb arugula salad: $1.99
½ avocado: 65 cents
1 lemon: 20 cents
1 red pepper: $1.15
1 box crimini mushrooms: $2.99
1 lb steamed Brussels sprouts: $1.99

Dessert: Fresh fruit
2 peaches: 98 cents
1 banana: 38 cents
Total cost: $17.55

NUTRITION
calories
1,979

macronutrients
carbohydrate: 404 grams
protein: 78.5 grams
fat: 30 grams
ratio: 75-12-13
fiber: 88.5 grams

micronutrients (as %DV)
vitamin A: 211
vitamin C: 1,124
vitamin D: 0
vitamin E: 128
vitamin B6: 539
vitamin B12: 0
calcium: 146
choline: 102
copper: 506
folate: 428
iron: 364
magnesium: 208
manganese: 411
niacin: 207
pantothenic acid: 324

phosphorus: 266
potassium: 237
riboflavin: 310
selenium: 222
sodium: 102
thiamin: 175
zinc: 147
water: 3.5 L (roughly 112 oz, or 14 cups)

At a very affordable price, this total plant diet supplies macronutrients in their proper proportion, a superabundance of fiber (nearly 90 grams), and well over 100 percent of the recommended intake of most essential nutrients (and in the case of vitamin C, over 1,000 percent!).

Maybe you have or are a teenager. Does this menu meet the nutritional needs of a growing guy or gal? Absolutely.

Teens have higher requirements for calcium and phosphorus than most adults. Specifically, teenage boys and girls require 1,300 mg of calcium per day. The above menu provides over 1,450 mg. Done.

The recommended phosphorus intake for teens is 1,250 mg. Again, the Paradigm plan exceeds this requirement, supplying over 1,850 mg of this important element.

Teenage boys require 11 mg of iron per day, more than males at other life stages. The Paradigm Diet supplies nearly 30 mg of iron, which meets the needs of all age groups and both genders, even pregnant females.

Perhaps you are pregnant or lactating. Congratulations. Your requirements for several nutrients are higher than otherwise. These include copper, iron, magnesium, manganese, phosphorus, potassium, selenium and zinc, as well as most vitamins. Most know that pregnant women have higher folate requirements (600 micrograms per day). Our sample diet provides 1,712 micrograms. Nearly three times the minimum amount!

And the 78.5 grams of protein provided by our sample meal plan meets everyone's requirement, whether you are child, adult, pregnant, lactating or exercising (but hopefully not being/doing all these at the same time!).[69] Are your fiber requirements met? Don't even ask. Obviously!

In addition, the 3.5 L of water contained in our menu meets the daily requirement for most people and does not even include a drop of liquid!

Our attempt is not to get caught up in individual nutrients and instead focus on a wholesome diet that provides more than enough of all nutrients, but now that we've started our analysis, we must see it through until the end, which raises the question.

Are there any nutrient requirements that plants do not fulfill?

Well, yes and no.

Our sample diet contains less than 100 percent of the recommended daily intake of 2 nutrients: vitamin B12 and vitamin D. (By comparison, 2,000 calories derived from equal parts tuna fish, whole wheat bread and raw almonds - 3 food groups we exclude - is deficient in 6 nutrients and has only 30 grams of fiber, 2 cups of water and zero vitamin C. Talk about starving your cells!)

Let's look more closely at these nutrients.

Vitamin B12

A water-soluble vitamin that your body is able to store for months or even years at a time, vitamin B12, also known as cobalamin, is needed for healthy nervous tissue and red blood cells. It is a trace vitamin, meaning very small amounts, measured in micrograms (one microgram equals one thousandth of a milligram), are required. Moreover, your body is able to recycle most of its B12, so deficiencies generally do not result except in diets that include absolutely no B12 for a period of decades, which is highly unlikely, if not impossible.[70]

Where does vitamin B12 come from? It is synthesized by bacteria. These critters are present both in the soil and in the intestinal tracts of animals, including humans. Food sources of vitamin B12 therefore include unwashed vegetables grown in rich soil, as well as animal tissue (meat products). However, because of the widespread use of pesticides and fertilizers (used in lieu of manure, which is B12-rich) and the cultural imperative to thoroughly wash our produce, there is likely little vitamin B12 on most fruits and vegetables by the time they meet your mouth.

The bacteria in your colon produce an abundance of B12. However, because B12 is absorbed higher up in your intestinal tract (at the level of the ileum, or third portion of the small intestine), the colonic source is less efficiently absorbed. Nevertheless, your body is able to use some of the B12 that intestinal bacteria produce, and evidence exists to suggest that bacteria higher up in your GI tract, at the level of the small intestine (the actual site of B12 absorption) also synthesize the vitamin in significant amounts.[71]

The foods richest in B12 are without exception animal foods, including liver, clams, fish and beef. Does this mean that meat eaters are unlikely to experience B12 deficiency? Not quite. One thing is ingesting B12. Another thing entirely is getting it into the bloodstream. Many people whose diets include large amounts of animal products, and therefore large amounts of vitamin B12, have low blood levels indicative of deficiency, as well as symptoms including fatigue and weakness. In fact, the National Institutes of Health estimates that as many as 15 percent of the general population is B12 deficient. In older adults, the prevalence is as high as 30 percent. In many instances, the cause is unknown, but most cases are due to atrophic gastritis and pernicious anemia, two disorders caused by damage to the stomach.[72]

Can meat eating damage the stomach? In a word, yes. Here's how. The **parietal cells** of the stomach are responsible for secreting a chemical known as *intrinsic factor*, which binds to B12 in food and helps your body absorb it in the small intestine. In many people with B12 deficiency, the parietal cells are damaged and fail to produce intrinsic factor. This condition is known as pernicious anemia. The parietal cells also produce *stomach acid*, so stomach acidity is decreased, a condition known as atrophic gastritis. Less stomach acid favors the growth of bacteria that use up the B12 for their own metabolic needs, leaving little left for your body to use.

So if B12 deficiency is due to damage to the cells lining your stomach, what causes the damage? Could it be that the injury suffered by the parietal cells is a direct product of years of excessive stomach acid, produced as a result of meat-heavy diets? Recall that the digestion of animal protein requires large amounts of stomach acid. Normally, the stomach produces mucus, which serves as a protective barrier from acid's corrosive effects. But over time, this barrier is penetrated and the parietal cells are damaged by the very chemical (acid) they secrete. Acid production is impaired, intrinsic factor diminishes and B12 deficiency inevitably ensues.

In short, the so-called best dietary source of B12 (meat) can with its high protein content actually cause the very damage that prevents B12 from ever meeting your bloodstream.

However, this is a matter of contention and additional research is required. Until then, you should obtain B12 in food, and for your best dietary source, look no further than nutritional yeast. As the name suggests, yeast is a nutritional powerhouse. It is made by fermenting microorganisms of the Saccharomyces family in sugar (often molasses), then drying the mixture.

Two tbsp (80 calories) of nutritional yeast provides 9 grams of protein and 5 grams of fiber, in addition to over 100 percent of the daily value of B12. (Not all brands of yeast contain B12, so before picking up a tub of the stuff, take a gander at the label.) Yeast is low in cost ($10 per lb), available at many markets, and its nutty, cheesy flavor will satisfy even the finicky palate. It can be added to salad, sprinkled over cooked vegetables and generally used in place of grated cheese.

NUTRITIONAL COMPARISON: YEAST AND CHEESE

<u>Parmesan cheese (3 tbsp)</u>
calories: 60
protein: 5.7 g
fat: 4 g
fiber: 0 g
Nutritional highlights (as %DV): 19% calcium, 11% phosphorus, less than 10% DV all other vitamins and minerals.

vs.

<u>Nutritional yeast (3 tbsp)</u>
calorie: 90
protein: 10.5 g
fat: 1 g
fiber: 5 g
Nutritional highlights (as %DV): 820% thiamine, 720% riboflavin, 370% niacin, 560% B6, 310% folic acid, 150% B12, 40% selenium, 25% zinc.

Vitamin D

A fat-soluble vitamin that acts like a hormone, vitamin D is principally known for its role in regulating calcium balance. Vitamin D also has strong anti-inflammatory properties, and it helps your immune system function properly, reducing your susceptibility to colds and cancer, for starters.[73] Additionally, there may be an association between low levels of vitamin D and depression.[74]

As with vitamin B12, animal products are the main dietary source of naturally-occurring vitamin D. In fact, the vitamin does not exist in plant foods, although fortified foods such as cereals and some varieties of mushrooms contain added D, as do milk products. If vitamin D does not occur in plants, where do herbivorous animals (cows) derive it from? One hint: Look up. (First, go outside, preferably before dark. And don't stare directly at it.) You got it. The sun. As with carbohydrate (and protein and fat, and many other nutrients) the ultimate source of vitamin D is the sun. If taken in adequate amounts, sunlight stimulates your skin to manufacture enough vitamin D to meet all your metabolic needs.

Sadly, most people are so afraid of getting too much sun, that many fail to get enough. Sun exposure is not synonymous with sun damage, and regular sun bathing should be seen as an integral component of a healthy life. What is enough sun? For the average person, **strong, direct sunlight over a large surface area (face, chest or back, arms or legs) that is exposed (no clothes) and unprotected (no sunscreen) for about 15 minutes, three times a week, between 10 AM and 3 PM**, should suffice. If you are darker-skinned or live far from the Equator, you may require more. During winter, you may wish to supplement with fortified mushrooms or a vitamin pill.

But whatever you do, do not obtain vitamin D from animal foods, which is like trying to strengthen your feet by shooting yourself in the foot. Allow us to explain. As mentioned, one of the major functions of vitamin D is calcium balance. Vitamin D helps your body absorb calcium, which is needed for strong bones (calcium is stored in the bone). Animal products, even those high in vitamin D and calcium (milk, fish), actually promote calcium loss and weakening of the bones. Here's how: Calcium is one of the major blood buffers, which means it is able to neutralize acids. So, when you eat animal protein, which is very acidic, your body pulls calcium from the bones, weakening them and causing tiny holes to form, a condition known as osteoporosis. This precious bone calcium is then excreted by your kidneys, which if you are dehydrated or have a family history can promote the development of kidney stones, one of the most painful conditions around. (Ouch!)

Because this seems counterintuitive, lets repeat it: Rather than strengthening your bones by increasing calcium absorption, vitamin D-rich animal foods such as dairy products, with their high protein content and despite their high calcium content, actually *leech* calcium from your bones, weakening them and causing more calcium to be excreted in the urine than these "calcium-rich" foods contain. The result is a net calcium loss, and porous bones that are increasingly susceptible to fracture with old age. *Ouch, my aching bones!*

So, get your vitamin D from yeast, or get out in the sun and make it yourself.

Antioxidant Vitamins (ACE)

We mention the antioxidants here because athletes may require larger doses of them. Exercise increases your metabolic rate and oxygen expenditure and causes you to produce more free radicals, so having more anti-oxidants on hand is a good idea. Vitamins A and C are obtainable in superabundance in a plant diet. One red pepper alone satisfies the recommended daily value of both, and eating a colorful assortment of fruits and vegetables makes getting large doses of these vitamins easy. You can meet the vitamin E requirement by emphasizing leafy green vegetables. Mustard greens, Swiss chard and turnip greens are excellent sources. Spinach is also an excellent source. In fact, 5 cups of boiled spinach, at a mere 200 calories, meets the daily requirement for most people. Unlike the vitamins A and C, however, this vitamin is harder to obtain in mega-doses, in food. If you are very active and feel you may require additional vitamin E, consider supplementation with an organic whole-food multivitamin, or simply **eat more steamed greens**. Nuts and oils are other sources, but as we've shown these foods are far too high in fat and too low in fiber and water to be deemed Paradigm. If you eat nuts, make them the exception rather than the rule. In other words, don't mistake them for a health food.

Getting back to our point. What was our point? Oh yes: available and affordable.

Not only does a diet predominately of sweets, greens, beans and seeds have availability and affordability in its corner. It is also

sustainable. In contrast to other diets that you try on like a spring skirt or a pair of soccer cleats, only to discard 'em next season, this style of eating – this *dietstyle*, if you will – is so easy and tasty, you can and likely will enjoy it indefinitely. As in, for the rest of your life. No eating loads of protein only to be left with bad breath, bad kidneys and fatigue. No wasting precious money on expensive, useless and potentially harmful pills, powders, shakes and supplements. No juicing lbs of carrots and tossing into the trash all that precious fiber (we tried this one: what a waste!). No ornate, overly-complicated cooking methods involving hours of toil over a hot stove...which brings us to our next criterion.

PROPERLY PREPARED

For a food to deserve the term *properly prepared*, it should be made in such a way that is easy, enhances taste and enhances or preserves nutrition.

Before we look into cooking methods, we must ask ourselves, do we need to cook at all? In other words, why isn't the Paradigm Diet entirely raw?

While raw vegetables should feature prominently in a healthy diet, there are drawbacks to an all-raw approach to food. Such a diet, while easy to prepare, would simply be too expensive and time-consuming, without supplying adequate calories. Raw vegetables are the lowest-calorie foods on the planet. One lb of raw spinach has 100 calories, some of which is used in the process of digestion (thermic effect of food, remember?). Also, some of those calories (about 40 percent, actually) are from fiber, which our body is incapable of deriving much if any energy from. With this in mind, the 100 calories in spinach, in terms of fuel we can use, is closer to 50. This means that if you ate exclusively raw vegetables, you'd need to consume nearly 4,000 calories a day to meet your energy needs, which is 80 lbs of spinach! Much of your day would be devoted to chewing your food, and much of your paycheck (or allowance) to paying for it.

While there are benefits to consuming a large proportion of food raw, excluding cooked food leaves out certain vegetables that are much tastier when placed over a flame. Remember, the most nutritionally dense foods are green vegetables, and most of them, including kale, broccoli, asparagus, Brussels sprouts and green beans, are more pleasing to the palate and can be consumed in far greater quantities if their fibers are softened and moistened with light cooking.

Some argue that cooking destroys the nutrients in food. It is true that cooking food in dry heat at high temperatures (higher than 212 degrees Fahrenheit), and for long periods of time destroys some nutrients, for example vitamin C and folic acid. However, cooking actually increases the bioavailability of certain nutrients, among them carotenoids such as beta-carotene, present for example in carrots, as well as lycopene, an antioxidant in tomatoes. And quickly cooking vegetables increases the amount of chlorophyll that your body can absorb. Chlorophyll is the blood of green vegetables, with a chemical structure closely resembling our own hemoglobin, the oxygen-carrying component of human blood. Lightly cooking food also reduces the content of goitrogens, oxalates and alkaloids present in certain foods, which may benefit sensitive individuals.[75] Additionally, cooking food kills harmful bacteria such as salmonella and E. coli which, in the modern era of factory farming, are increasingly present in food.

Of course, not all cooking methods are created equal.

When food is steamed, boiled or sautéed, the temperature is fixed at the temperature of boiling water. Unlike dry heat methods such as broiling, roasting and baking, which cause food to dry out, turn brown and form toxic compounds, using water in cooking adds to the moisture present in foods and prevents the temperature from rising to unhealthful levels. Boiling, steaming or sautéing vegetables allows you to preserve or even enhance their nutritional benefits while you consume much larger portions in fewer mouthfuls. This is important given the low calorie content of greens. Consider that 2.5 cups of boiled spinach has as many calories (100) as 15 cups of raw spinach. And per cup, boiled spinach has over 5 times as much vitamin C as raw spinach.

What about the enzymes?! We hear you scream. Good one. We hear this question all the time, especially from raw foodists, who claim that humans require the digestive enzymes present in fruits and vegetables in order to properly assimilate the nutrients in these foods.

This is not the case.

Yes, it is true that fruits and vegetables contain an abundance of enzymes. Enzymes are proteins and make up a large portion of the protein content of vegetables such as spinach, which as we mentioned derives nearly half of its calories from protein. But these enzymes are specific to the fruit or vegetable itself, catalyzing reactions necessary to the survival of the plants in question, not us.

While it is true that cooking deactivates the enzymes present in plants, the acid environment of the stomach, with a pH as low as 1 or 2 (very, very acidic!) can denature enzymes even more quickly than cooking. But preserving the function of enzymes is irrelevant, because as enzymes they do us no service. What we need to concern ourselves with is the amino acid components of these enzymes, which our body is able to use as building blocks for our own proteins and enzymes. And though cooking food and exposing it to stomach acid denatures enzymes and interferes with their function as enzymes, it does not destroy them. The amino acids that make up enzymes are available to your body whether you cook your meal or eat it raw.

As we covered, your body is fully equipped with a sufficient amount of digestive enzymes (proteases, amylases, lipases, among others) to handle the relatively small load of protein, fat and carbohydrates present in fruits and vegetables. Moreover, many of the calories in fruits and vegetables are free sugar molecules (glucose and fructose) and do not require any enzyme activity whatsoever.

Yes, animals thrive on diets consisting of raw foods. But most humans do not have the time or the patience to chew food as thoroughly as a cow or ape. And in an exclusively raw diet, such assiduous chewing is required to fully pulverize the cell walls of plants and make them available for assimilation. Cooking aids digestion by doing the work that our teeth once did, and that the molars of animals still do. Of course we are talking about lightly cooking vegetables, in other words preparing them *al dente,* to borrow from the Italians. Overcooking veggies, or exposing them to chemicals and oils, turns them into empty-calorie mush that neither pleases the palate nor does a body good.

Of all the cooking methods, microwaving food may be the most harmful. Microwaving food can expose the user to harmful radiation that may manifest as *microwave sickness,* whose symptoms include night sweats, insomnia, headaches, depression, nausea, swollen lymph nodes and impaired thinking. If you have a microwave, don't use it. Or better yet, lose it.

Cooking methods to LOSE
Microwaving
Frying
Sautéing in oil
Grilling
Roasting
Broiling
Baking

Cooking methods to USE
Boiling
Steaming
Sautéing in water or vegetable broth

Of course you are encouraged to include as many raw fruits and vegetables into your diet as you can – for example, by blending fresh fruit and leafy greens for breakfast, having raw fruit for lunch and starting dinner off with a large raw vegetable salad. Then, make judicious use of the healthiest forms of cooking to expand nutrient density and absorption of plant protein. In the next chapter we will explore these cooking methods individually.

ENVIRONMENTALLY FRIENDLY

In order to determine the environmental effects of consuming plant foods, we must examine the land acreage, water supply and fuel expenditure used to produce them. Then we can compare their effect on the environment to that of other foods.[76]

Land acreage: Let us say that you were given 2.5 acres of land to produce food for your loved ones. For the athletes in the house, this is about 2 football fields. If you used this land to produce a vegetable (say, cabbage), you could feed over 20 people. If you used the land to produce wheat, 15 people could eat their fill. However, if chicken or milk were your product, then you could supply the calorie needs of only yourself and a loved one (two people). If you used the land to produce eggs or beef, which in turn would need grains and grass, you would only have enough food for yourself. The rest of your neighborhood would starve. Doesn't this sound an awful lot like what is going on in the world today?

Energy: To produce 1 calorie of protein from soybeans, 2 calories of fossil fuel (coal, oil, natural gas) are required. By contrast, one calorie of protein from beef requires 54 calories of fossil fuel. This is over 25 times the energy expenditure. In a given day, the amount of greenhouse-warming carbon gas released by a typical car is 3 kilograms. Seventy-five kilograms of carbon gas are released by clearing and burning enough rainforest to produce beef for one hamburger, or 25 times as much. Perhaps if you were forbidden from driving your car for a month and made to hoof it or hitch it each time you ate a hamburger, you might reconsider your next visit to Boogers R Us.

Water supply: The production of 1 lb of lettuce requires over 20 gallons of water. One lb of apples needs 50 gallons of water to supply its metabolic needs. Sound like a lot? Not by comparison to animal foods. One lb of chicken uses up over 800 gallons of water. Pork consumes twice as much, or over 1,600 gallons. The number of gallons of water used to produce 1 lb of beef? Over 5,000 gallons.

As you can see, beef uses up a large portion of our water supply, more gallons per lb than the other foods combined! The real cause of the water shortage is in the meat. In fact, _1 lb of beef wastes enough water to provide a person with a 7-minute hot shower every day for a year._

In these sad times of water shortage, avoiding showering can diminish your enjoyment of life and make you stinky. Instead, simply eat less meat – with a target consumption of zero.

And who eats the world's beef? None more so than the United States. Though the US is home to only 4 percent of the world's population, Americans consume nearly 25 percent of the beef on the planet. In other words, Americans chow 8 times the amount of cow as citizens of other countries.

And this prodigious beef consumption takes a powerful economic toll that each and every meat eater would deeply feel were it not for government subsidizing of the meat and dairy industries, which receive nearly 75 percent of all federal monies given to food manufacturers. Were it not for this subsidizing, the price of that $2 fast food hamburger you pay without giving it much thought would total as much as $200.00,[77] likely more than anyone in her right mind would pay for toxic flesh. Federal generosity in the case of meat explains why many animal products, at $2 to $4 per lb, are less expensive than fruits and vegetables, which receive almost no government funding.

It does not seem unrelated then, that over 50 percent of the children in some 3rd world countries are so *under*fed and *under*weight that their health suffers, which corresponds almost exactly to the percentage of adults in the US who are so *over*fed and *over*weight as to have health problems.

Americans are feeding themselves to death with foods that consume the environment, and as a result, other Earthlings (animals, children) are suffering and dying.

How to end world hunger? Simple as 1, 2, 3. Stop. Eating Meat. Put another way: Eat. More. Greens. And beans. And sweets. And seeds.

In fact, the United Nations issued a report in June 2010 urging that *a global shift towards a vegan diet is vital to save the world from hunger, fuel impacts and the worst impacts of climate change.*[78] This is the United Nations speaking, not some tree-hugging hairy-legged militant vegan. The UN is an unbiased organization existing for the common good of humanity. Can recommendations get any clearer or more concise? This is black and white, people. Meat is black (bad). Plants are white. And blue. And green. And every other color of the rainbow, these colors signifying the presence of a variety of potent anti-oxidants that keep you young, energetic and alive.

A plant diet is nonviolent, and as we have shown, it is in accordance with our anatomical and physiological design. It is also in accordance with Nature. Choosing plant food over other foods encourages the cultivation of fields, herbs and trees, which makes the world a greener place.

As you may remember from biology class, green plants contain chlorophyll. By the process of photosynthesis plants use chlorophyll to convert the sun's energy into fuel (the sugars in their leaves, roots and fruits), while cleansing the atmosphere of carbon dioxide and replacing it with the oxygen we need to breathe.

PHOTOSYNTHESIS

$$6CO_2 + 6H_2O \text{ -----> } C_6H_{12}O_6 + 6O_2$$
carbon dioxide + water ----> sugar + oxygen

Green plants supply our lungs with air and our bodies with energy. Together we exist in a symbiotic relationship, sympathetic and mutually beneficial. Without trees and their leaves, seeds, roots and fruits, we would have neither sugar nor oxygen. In short, we could neither move nor breathe. In short, we'd cease to exist. We'd go extinct. Yikes! How do we show our gratitude to green plants? By cutting them down, leveling forests to make way for cattle grazing. We exist in an antagonistic relationships with animals, whom we hunt down, coop up and subject to violent abuses only to die of animal food-related diseases ourselves. But you know this already. Let's look at the bright side:

Plants feed the planet and the planet feeds us. To go green is to give back to the planet that gives to you. Plants. Planet. People. Peace. Paradigm. See a trend here?

UNREFINED, UNPROCESSED AND WHOLE

With the exception of nutritional yeast and basic condiments, the Paradigm Foods are whole, natural foods that appear on the plate just as they do on the plant.

Processed foods, including supplements (energy bars, protein powders and fortified foods including breads and breakfast cereals) lump together a mishmash of different ingredients, strip away the fiber and essential fats, put back a small amount of a few vitamins, dehydrate the whole and label it nutritious. Even so-called *superfoods* pay no mind to the laws of food combination. Frequently you find protein (soy, whey, casein, hemp) combined with starch (rice, wheat, oats) and mixed with concentrated fats (nuts, seeds, chocolate), possibly with some form of genetically-modified corn (starch, syrup) mixed in. Talk about a gastrointestinal nightmare! These man-made foods (*Frankenfoods*, as they are sometimes called) do not exist in nature. We did not evolve eating them. They are foreign to the system, which must work overtime to process them and eventually goes kaput! The result: indigestion, fatigue, weight gain and just plain feeling like crap!

Convenience items such as vending machine snacks are even worse. These *refined* foods come in two classes. The first (baked goods, pastries) are made of grains that have been stripped of their nutrients and fibers (in other words, refined) until only their sugars remain. This helps to increase shelf life, because so devoid of nutrition white bread and other refined grains do not even appeal to mold. They are fashioned into flour and turned into all sorts of cookies, brownies, donuts, muffins and chips. The second class, candies, are concentrated corn sugar that is then colored, flavored and shaped into bite-sized recipes for diabetes and dental decay.

Packaged foods may be convenient, but they are *deleterious*. Fresh fruit, on the other hand, is convenient and *nutritious*. It comes in Nature's package, be it peel or rind, and palm-sized. A sun-kissed handful of sweet gold.

Processed foods may contain added vitamins and minerals, or they may not, but either way these piecemeal foods are difficult to digest, and a few extra nutrients do not change this. Besides, no amount of added nutrients can approach the total amount of nourishment existing in whole plants. If you believe you require more nutrition outside of what is offered by a total whole-food plant diet, you are likely being duped by the supplement industry. If you are still fixated on more nutrition and a nutritional analysis verifies deficiencies, add an organic whole-food multivitamin to your morning shake. It fortifies your diet without the extra calories, fat and poor food combinations. Or better still, nutritional yeast has the additional benefit of fiber and great taste.

Is the Paradigm Diet extreme or limiting? Ironically, the ones who ask this are those who eat chicken at most meals. How is meat eating not boring? Where animal protein is concerned, you are limited to a few choices: beef, pig, fish, fowl, eggs and milk derivatives. There may be a few others, but not nearly as many as the nearly one hundred easy to come by, easy to prepare, delicious and nutritious fruits and vegetables waiting to be discovered and enjoyed at your next meal.

So what are you waiting for?

THE PARADIGM FOODS

Sweets: apples, apricots, bananas, blackberries, blueberries, cantaloupe, cherries, dates, figs, grapefruit, grapes, lemons, limes, kiwi, mango, nectarines, melons, oranges, papayas, peaches, pears, persimmons, pineapples, plums, prunes, raisins, raspberries, strawberries, tangerines, watermelons

Greens: artichokes, asparagus, beet greens, bok choy, broccoli, Brussels sprouts, cabbage, celery, collard greens, kale, lettuce, mustard greens, snap peas, spinach, string beans, Swiss chard, turnip greens, zucchini, herbs (basil, cilantro, dill, oregano, parsley)

Beans: adzuki beans, black beans, black-eyed peas, chickpeas, kidney beans, lentils, lima beans, mung beans, navy beans, pinto beans, soybeans, white beans

Other vegetables: avocados, beets, bell peppers, carrots, cauliflower, cucumbers, eggplant, garlic, mushrooms, olives, onions, potatoes, pumpkins, radishes, squash, sweet potatoes, tomatoes, water chestnuts, yams

Seeds: chia, flax

THE PARADIGM FOODS: APPLES TO ZUCCHINI[79]

In case the only vegetables you're used to eating are French fries and maybe the occasional carrots, corn and peas, or even if you're a veritable connoisseur, here is a brief introduction to the Paradigm Foods.

For each item, we list the proper cooking method, as well as those nutrients it is *high* in. To qualify as being *high*, a given food does not have to smoke pot; rather, it must contain at least 25 percent of the nutrient in question, per 100 calories. For example, 100 calories of asparagus contains 75 percent of the daily value of vitamin C and is therefore *high* in vitamin C. Naturally high, no prescription required.

GREENS

asparagus: the aristocrat of vegetables, asparagus is high in vitamin K, folate, vitamin C, vitamin A, thiamin, riboflavin, manganese, fiber and vitamin B6; sauté asparagus for 5 minutes

beet greens: similar in taste and texture to spinach and Swiss chard, beet greens are high in vitamin K, vitamin A, vitamin C, potassium, manganese, riboflavin, magnesium, copper, thiamin, fiber, calcium and iron; quick boil beet greens for 1 minute

bok choy: a mild-flavored member of the cabbage family, bok choy is high in vitamin A, calcium, vitamin C, vitamin B6 and manganese; enjoy both the stalks and the leafy green portions by sautéing for 5 minutes

broccoli: this popular cruciferous vegetable is high in vitamin C, vitamin K, vitamin A, folate, fiber, manganese, potassium, vitamin B6 and riboflavin; steam broccoli for 5 minutes

Brussels sprouts: a hearty cruciferous vegetable from northern Europe, Brussels sprouts are high in vitamin K, vitamin C, folate, vitamin A, manganese and fiber; slice them in half and steam for 5 minutes

cabbage: enjoyed for thousands of years in Russia, Germany and China, red cabbage and green cabbage are high in vitamin K, vitamin

C, fiber, manganese and vitamin B6; as with bok choy, sauté for 5 minutes in vegetable broth

celery: for centuries enjoyed by the Greeks and Romans both as a flavor enhancer in soups and raw as a crunchy snack, celery is high in vitamin K, vitamin C, potassium, folate, fiber, molybdenum, manganese, B6 and calcium; enjoy it raw, or sauté for 5 minutes

collard greens: smoky and meaty, this Southern specialty is high in vitamin K, vitamin A, vitamin C, manganese, folate, calcium, fiber, potassium, and B6; slice them thin and enjoy both the stem and the leaves after steaming for 5 minutes

green peas: a Biblical vegetable, green peas are high in vitamin K, manganese, vitamin C and fiber; *garden peas* need to be shelled before cooking, while *snow peas* can be eaten in the shell/pod – both varieties should be sautéed for 3 minutes; *sugar snap peas* are crunchier and sweeter and can be eaten raw and in the pod

kale: another cruciferous vegetable enjoyed thousands of years the world over, kale is high in vitamin K, vitamin A, vitamin C, manganese, fiber, copper, calcium and B6; steam kale for 5 minutes along with other greens (broccoli, collards)

lettuce: depicted on the tombs of ancient Egyptians and a good luck charm to the Chinese, lettuce is high in vitamin K, vitamin A, vitamin C, folate, manganese, chromium, potassium, molybdenum, fiber, thiamin, iron, riboflavin, phosphorus and calcium; enjoy all the luscious varieties (red leaf, butterhead, leaf lettuce, Romaine, arugula, mixed greens) raw

mustard greens: a pungent member of the cruciferous family, with a very intense flavor, mustard greens are high in vitamin K, vitamin A, vitamin C, folate, manganese, vitamin E, fiber, calcium, potassium, B6, protein, copper phosphorus, iron , riboflavin and magnesium; sauté this powerhouse green for 3 minutes

spinach: popularized by Popeye, spinach is rich in vitamin K, vitamin A, manganese, folate, magnesium, iron, vitamin C, vitamin B2, calcium, potassium, vitamin B6, fiber, copper, thiamin and protein; enjoy it raw, or boiled for 1 minute.

string beans: also called green beans, string beans are high in vitamin K, vitamin C, manganese, vitamin A and fiber; enjoy them raw or steam them for 5 minutes, but do not overcook

Swiss chard: praised by Aristotle, Swiss chard is high in vitamin K, vitamin A, vitamin C, magnesium, manganese, potassium, iron, vitamin E, fiber, copper, calcium and riboflavin; boil Swiss chard with spinach and beet greens (put chard in first, wait 1 minute, add beet greens, wait 1 minute, add spinach, wait 1 minute and serve)

turnip greens: resembling mustard greens in flavor, turnip greens are high in vitamin A, vitamin C, manganese, calcium, copper, fiber and vitamin E; sauté them with mustard greens in vegetable broth

SWEETS

apples: the fruit of knowledge is rich in antioxidants; try all the lovely varieties of apples, including Red Delicious, Fuji, Gala, Golden Delicious, Granny Smith, McIntosh, Jonathan and crab apples

apricots: one of the first fruits of summer, apricots are high in Vitamin A and vitamin C

bananas: called the fruit of paradise, bananas are high in B6 and one of the best sources of potassium

berries: enjoy all the lovely varieties: black, blue, boysenberries, raspberries, cherries, cranberries and strawberries; simply bursting with nutrition

cantaloupe: refreshingly rich and aromatic, cantaloupe is high in vitamin C, vitamin A and potassium

dates: a Biblical fruit, dates are a concentrated source of simple sugar to provide you with quick energy and satisfy even the stubbornest of sweet teeth; medjool are our favorite

figs: another Biblical fruit, the luscious, sweet-tasting fig is a universal symbol of virility; choose raw over dried, though both are good

grapefruit: the slightly larger cousin of the orange is tangy and high in vitamin C

grapes and raisins: these sweet bursts of simple sugar are perfect on a hot day; buy organic

lemons and limes: tart and acidic yet refreshing, these tangy citrus twins are high in vitamin C; blend into a smoothie, add to your fruit salad, or squeeze atop a salad

kiwi: this wonder fruit is high in vitamin C; most peel before eating, but the skin is high in fiber and should be tried

mango: this tropical fruit is sun-filled nectar; high in vitamin A and vitamin C

nectarines and peaches: don't miss the low-calorie refreshing burst of vitamins A and C and fiber that these palm-sized blessings offer

oranges: easy to pack (and plant) and fun to eat, oranges are high in vitamin C; cut up 10 oranges, mix into a bowl, and enjoy for lunch on a bright sunny day

papayas: these luscious fruits the color of the sun are high in vitamin C and folate; spritz with lemon for added tang

persimmons: the fruit of the gods, persimmons are widely available around Halloween; try the crispy fuyu variety and bite into it just like an apple

pineapples: exceptionally sweet and juicy, pineapples are high in manganese and vitamin C; opt for locally-grown fruits, which are more flavorful and nutritious

plums and prunes: these ancient fruits have the antioxidant profile to keep you eternally youthful; opt for plums whenever possible, and have prunes with water

watermelons: arguably the most refreshing fruit of them all, watermelon has a low glycemic load and high levels of vitamins A and C

BEANS

adzuki beans: easier to digest than most beans, adzukis are slightly sweet and a suitable substitute for kidney beans; simmer 1 cup of beans in 3 cups of water for 1.5 hours or until soft – no soaking necessary; also available canned

black beans: high in molybdenum, folate and fiber, the rich, earthy flavor of black beans balances the spice of even the spiciest dish; soak overnight and simmer 1 cup of beans in 3 cups of water for 1.5 hours; available canned

black-eyed peas: a good source of selenium, black-eyed peas are easily digested; soak and simmer 1 cup of peas in 4 cups of water for 1.5 hours; canned varieties available

canellini beans: also called white kidney beans, they taste like great northern but are longer and more plump; soak and simmer 1 cup in 3 cups water for 1.5 hours or buy canned; throw them onto a salad

chickpeas: also called garbanzos, they are high in molybdenum, manganese and folate; soak and simmer 1 cup in 4 cups water for 3 hours, or buy canned

great northern beans: soak and simmer 1 cup of these canellini look-alikes in 3 cups water for 2 hours, or buy canned

kidney beans: sweet and subtle, kidneys are great substitutions for meat dishes; high in molybdenum and folate; soak and simmer 1 cup in 4 cups water for 1.5 hours, or buy canned

lentils: the king legume, lentils are high in molybdenum, folate and fiber; do not require soaking and have short cooking times; simmer 1 cup in 2 cups water for half an hour

lima beans: buttery and starchy, lima beans are delicious cooked with herbs; high in molybdenum and fiber; soak and simmer 1 cup in 4 cups water for 1.5 hours; canned varieties hard to find but available

mung beans: a major feature of Indian dishes and Chinese cuisine, they are easy to digest, though they do not hold their shape; simmer 1 cup in 4 cups water for 1.5 hours; or try sprouting

navy beans: great with kale, navy beans are delicious soaked and simmered in 4 cups water for 2.5 hours

peas (split peas): this member of the legume family has been cultivated for over 20,000 years and is high in molybdenum and fiber; no soaking required; simmer 1 cup in 3 cups water for 30 minutes

pinto beans: this Mexican favorite, pintos are high in molybdenum, folate and fiber; should be soaked overnight and simmered for 2 hours in 4 cups water; are also great refried, but do not use oil or lard: simply mash in a pan and add vegetable broth and onion until soft

soybeans: this sweet, nutty bean is also high in fat and requires lengthy cooking times; soak in refrigerator and cook for at least 3 hours in 3 cups of water, until soft

tofu: this processed soy product, also known as the cheese of Asia, is high in manganese and iron; eat sparingly as tofu is high in fat, and buy only organic as soy is a common genetically-modified food

SEEDS

chia: grown in Mexico, this dietary staple of the Aztecs and Mayans is high in fiber and omega-3 fatty acids; enjoy 1 tbsp daily, mixed into water or blended in a smoothie

flax: this earthy and warm seed is high in omega-3 fatty acids, manganese and fiber; grind just prior to using and enjoy in a smoothie or sprinkled over salads

RAINBOW VEGETABLES

avocados: a part of human history for over 10,000 years, this tropical fruit with its smooth, buttery flavor is an excellent addition to any dish; enjoy an avocado a day

beets: this root vegetable related to the carrot and distinguished by its vibrant red color is high in folate and manganese; cut into pieces and steam for 15 minutes

bell peppers: versatile and colorful, bell peppers are high in vitamin C, vitamin A, vitamin B6 and fiber; enjoy them raw or sauté in broth for 7 minutes

carrots: not just for silly rabbits, this root vegetable is high in vitamin A, vitamin K, vitamin C and fiber; eat raw or steam for 5 minutes

cauliflower: broccoli's albino cousin, cauliflower is high in vitamin C, vitamin K, folate, fiber, B6, manganese and omega-3 fatty acids

cucumbers: crunchy, refreshing and hydrating, cucumbers are high in vitamin C, molybdenum, vitamin A, potassium, manganese, folate and fiber (not bad for being 95 percent water); slice, salt and enjoy

eggplant: originally found in the Indian wild, eggplant is high in fiber and potassium; slice into cubes and sauté for 7 minutes; no need to peel if you buy organic

garlic: this hotly pungent bulb fueled the building of the pyramids; it's high in manganese, B6 and C; chop it up and add it to salads and cooked dishes

mushrooms: the immortal food, mushrooms are savory and nutritious; high in selenium, riboflavin, copper, niacin, B5, potassium, phosphorus, zinc, manganese, thiamin and B6; varieties include button, Shiitake, portabella and crimini or brown, which are especially nutritious; eat raw with nutritional yeast and salt or slice and sauté for 7 minutes

olives: one of the oldest foods, olives are a symbol of peace and wisdom; noted for their iron, vitamin E, fiber and copper content; buy saltwater-soaked varieties and add to any dish for flavor and satisfaction

onions: used as currency to fund the building of ancient monuments, onions are high in chromium and vitamin C; many varieties exist and include storage onions (yellow, Spanish, red, white, boiling) which are pungent, and spring/summer onions (Walla Walla, Vidalia and Maui Sweet) which can be eaten raw in salads; green onions and scallions are another option

potatoes: this tuber is a dietary staple in many countries; dozens of varieties exist; we recommend red potatoes; cut into 1/2-inch cubes and steam for 10 minutes

radishes: this root vegetable is high in fiber, vitamin C and copper; enjoy it raw and seasoned

squash: highly regarded by Native Americans, winter squash is high in vitamin A, vitamin C, potassium, fiber and manganese; varieties include butternut, acorn, spaghetti squash and sugar pumpkins; peel, cube and steam for 7 minutes

sweet potatoes: cultivated in Peru 10,000 years back and brought to the New World by Mr. Columbus in 1492, sweet potatoes are high in vitamin A, vitamin C and manganese; many varieties exist, including yams which are really not yams; cut into cubes and steam for 7 minutes

tomatoes: this vegetable fruit is high in vitamins C, A and K, and the minerals molybdenum, potassium and manganese; varieties include cherry tomatoes, greens, plums, heirlooms and slicing tomatoes; enjoy them raw, canned or sautéed for 5 minutes

zucchini: the summer squash, as it is also called, is high in manganese, vitamin C, magnesium, vitamin A, fiber, potassium, copper and folate; it has edible skin, soft seeds and a high water content, making it easier to cook than winter varieties; simply dice and sauté in broth for 3 minutes

HERBS AND SPICES

cocoa: cocoa powder is surprisingly low in calories (15 per tbsp) and high in antioxidants; 1 tbsp has 5,850 antioxidant (ORAC) units (equivalent to 1 cup of blueberries)

cayenne/red chili pepper: hot and feisty, chili powder is high in vitamin A, vitamin C, manganese, B6 and fiber; increase the flavor and impact of any dish, including smoothies; (1,500 ORAC/tbsp)

cinnamon: one of the oldest spices, cinnamon is high in manganese, fiber, iron and calcium; add it to smoothies, or sprinkle atop a fruit salad (18,500 ORAC/tbsp)

basil: a token of love, basil is high in vitamin K, iron, calcium, vitamin A, fiber, manganese, magnesium and vitamin C; enjoy it fresh in any dish; sprinkled dried varieties over vegetables (4,500 ORAC/tbsp dried)

cilantro: also called Chinese parsley, cilantro is high in vitamin K and vitamin A; enjoy it fresh or dried

dill: a sign of wealth, this aromatic and sweet herb is high in iron, manganese and calcium; use fresh or dried

mint: pleasantly warm, fresh, aromatic and sweet, with a cool aftertaste, mint leaves are high in vitamin A, vitamin C, calcium, iron, manganese, copper and magnesium; wonderful blended in smoothies

stevia: a sweat-leaf herb native to the Americas, stevia is processed into powder and used as a no-calorie sweetener

turmeric: this prized spice is high in manganese, iron, B6 and fiber; add to any dish to enrich the color and flavor (11,500 ORAC/tbsp)

WEEKLY SHOPPING CHECKLIST

[ ] 3 lbs leafy greens: one lettuce, two types of cooking greens (spinach, kale, chard)

[ ] 3 lbs solid greens: example broccoli, asparagus, Brussels sprouts

[ ] 3 lbs non-green vegetables: eggplant, mushrooms, cauliflower

[ ] 2 spicy vegetables: onion, garlic

[ ] 2 lbs vegetable fruits: bell peppers, cucumber

[ ] 2 fatty fruits: olives, avocado

[ ] 2 juicy fruits: watermelon, cantaloupe

[ ] 2 concentrated fruits: bananas, dates

[ ] 2 frozen fruits: blueberries, strawberries

[ ] 2 lbs of lemons

[ ] 6 cans of beans (kidney, garbanzo, black)

[ ] 2 bags of potatoes (red and sweet)

[ ] 2 cans of diced tomatoes (ingredients: tomatoes, water, salt)

[ ] 1 tub of nutritional yeast

[ ] 1 package flax or chia seeds

[ ] Condiments: mustard, hot sauce, soy sauce, olive tapenade

[ ] Spices: black pepper, cacao, cayenne, cinnamon, chili flakes

[ ] Herbs: basil, cilantro, dill, oregano, stevia

COURSE THREE: THE PARADIGM APPLIED

As we have shown, the healthiest diet on the planet consists exclusively of plants. Each species has its characteristic food. For humans, this food is plants. Fruits, vegetables, and legumes (beans, peas, lentils) are designed by nature to be our exclusive food. Just as we breathe only air, and are best suited to drink fresh water, plants are our perfect food.

The Paradigm Diet is a raw and lightly cooked whole-food, plant diet, high in carbohydrate (80 percent of calories), with sufficient protein (10 percent) and fat (10 percent) and enough water and fiber to ensure optimal gastrointestinal function.

On a 2,000 calorie diet, this translates to 400 grams of carbohydrates (1600 calories), 50 grams of protein (200 calories), and 20-25 grams of fat (200 calories), with 50 grams of fiber, at least.

Remember our *Paradigm Pyramid.*

SEEDS
BEANS
SWEETS
GREENS

PARADIGM PYRAMID

Each day strive to consume:

2

tbsp of seeds

4

glasses of fresh water

6

servings of starch (beans, bananas, squash, potatoes)

700 calories

8

servings of fruits

800 calories

10

servings of vegetables, vegetable fruits and fatty fruits

500 calories

If you are very active or actively growing and require additional calories, simply eat more of the same.

SERVING SIZES

Fruit

One medium, or 1 cup

Example of 8 servings: a breakfast smoothie with 3 cups watermelon (3 servings), 2 bananas (2), 1 cup berries (1); a piece of fruit before lunch and after dinner (2); for dessert, have more fruit if desired

Vegetables

For most vegetables, 1 lb equals 3 cups equals 3 servings equals 100 calories, raw or cooked.

One serving is 1 cup of vegetables, 1 whole vegetable fruit (cucumber, pepper, tomato) or 150 calories of fatty fruit (half of an avocado or 15 olives)

Example of 10 servings: 1 lb raw lettuce (3 servings), 1 lb steamed broccoli (3), 1 bell pepper (1), 1 cucumber (1), 1 tomato (1), ½ avocado (1).

These 10 servings may be consumed in the same meal. Say, at dinner if you've eaten only fruit all day, which we highly recommend!

For dinner, simply toss steamed broccoli into a big, colorful salad. Or, start with a large plate of assorted raw veggies, and follow this with a bowl of beans and broccoli.

Beans/Potatoes

One can of beans equals 3 servings equals 1.5 cups. One medium potato or sweet potato is 1 serving.

Work to as much as 1 to 2 cans of beans per day; start with one-half a can a day. Eat 1 to 2 potatoes per day.

The USDA is now recommending that for dinner, half of the plate should be devoted to fruits and vegetables, while the other half contains a mixture of protein and starches.[80]

The Paradigm dinner follows these guidelines exactly. Half the calories derive from green vegetables and vegetable fruits, while the other half are in the form of starches such as potatoes and squash, as well as beans, which are high in protein.

BRINGING IT ALL TOGETHER

To incorporate this "dietstyle" as quickly and efficiently as possible, we need to touch on a few topics. These are **cleaning out the kitchen, going grocery shopping** and **properly preparing food.**

ONE: CLEAN OUT YOUR KITCHEN

If you live with others and are reinventing your diet all on your lonesome, make sure to reserve a shelf in the pantry, a place on the counter and some space in the refrigerator to call your own. Families and those who live alone can use more or all of the kitchen space.

Then, do these three things:

Step One: Introduce More Produce

Fill your kitchen with these:

* 3 leafy greens: one lettuce, two cooking greens (spinach, kale, chard)
* 3 solid greens: broccoli, asparagus, green beans
* 3 non-green vegetables: eggplant, mushrooms, cauliflower
* 2 spicy vegetables: onion, garlic
* 2 vegetable fruits: bell peppers, cucumber
* 2 fatty fruits: olives, avocado
* 2 juicy fruits: watermelon, cantaloupe
* 2 concentrated fruits: bananas, dates
* 2 frozen fruits: blueberries, strawberries
* 2 frozen veggies: broccoli/cauliflower mix, and stir-fry
* 2 lbs of lemons

Step Two: Remove Deadly Foods

Start eliminating these: meat, eggs, dairy, baked goods, sweets, oils and processed, refined, packaged goods. Included in your *to toss* list is most anything that carries a label other than fruits, vegetables, beans or condiments, especially if the label contains corn, flour or trans fats. Seize foods with ingredients such as *unbleached wheat flour, high fructose corn syrup* or *partially-hydrogenated vegetable oil* and give them or throw them away. Better tossed in the *waste* than worn on your *waist* (or hips or thighs), we say.

Step Three: Replace Dead Foods with These

* 3 cans of beans (kidney, garbanzo, black)
* 2 cans of diced tomatoes (ingredients: tomatoes, water, salt)

* 1 tub of nutritional yeast
* An assortment of healthy condiments: mustard, hot sauce, soy sauce alternative, olive tapenade
* Assorted spices: chili flakes, cayenne, turmeric, pepper

TWO: GROCERY SHOPPING

Shop with a list in hand. Use the one provided a couple pages back. Spend most of your time in the produce section. Think of yourself as a kid in a candy store and choose as many colorful, sweet fruits as your stomach will hold. Remember, most of it is water and fiber. Shop twice weekly if you can, buying only enough fresh food to last 3 to 5 days, and as much frozen and canned items as you wish.

THREE: PROPERLY PREPARING FOOD

As we have shown, plant foods fulfill the requirements for most major vitamins and minerals, while adequately supplying protein and fat and doubling or tripling your fiber needs, at a cost of under $15 per day.

But all this means little if the food is not properly prepared.

The healthiest way to eat is to prepare your own food. Say it again. The healthiest way to eat is to prepare my own food. Say it aloud. The healthiest way to eat is to prepare my own food. Tell a friend. The healthiest way to eat is to prepare your own food.

Got it?

Preparing your own food is nutritious, delicious, cost-effective and convenient. By becoming your own personal chef, you control exactly what goes into your meal. No MSG, GMO or partially-hydrogenated anything. No empty calories or hidden oils. Better still, no boogers, poop or pubic hairs allowed.

Preparing food for yourself and for your loved ones is easy to do. All of the dishes you'll soon learn to prepare can be made in **under 10 minutes**, and all revolve around the same **three easy cooking methods**: boiling, steaming and sautéing in water or broth. You will need the following cookware:

- 12-inch stainless steel skillet or wok for sautéing.
- 4-quart stainless steel steamer for steaming and boiling

THE COOKING METHODS[81]

We love to cook, but like most people, we'd rather not spend our whole lives in the kitchen.

Luckily, the healthiest forms of cooking - sautéing, steaming and boiling - are also the quickest and involve the least amount of cleanup. As all three methods use moisture, they require a temperature that does not exceed 212 degrees Fahrenheit and thus preserve much of the nutrient content in food while improving its digestibility. By contrast, oven-based and stovetop cooking methods range from 350 to 450 degrees Fahrenheit, which makes burning and charring food likely. This is a recipe for cancer. Not on our menu.

For best results, always use the method of cooking most suited to a particular vegetable. For example, boiling rather than steaming spinach reduces its acidity and improves its flavor. While it is certainly nutritious to eat steamed spinach, it is not as tasty, and it gives you gritty teeth.

BOILING

Cooking vegetables in boiling water is the easiest of all methods, as it involves the shortest cooking times, no preparation and zero cleanup. Boiling maximizes the flavor and the nutritional benefits of spinach and bean sprouts, for example. Take special care not to exceed the recommended time limit, as nutrient loss increases dramatically with longer cooking times. For this reason, consider using a timer.

To boil vegetables, fill your pot three-quarters full with water and bring to a rapid boil. Then, add your vegetables, but do not cover. Start the timer the moment the vegetables come in contact with the water. After a minute give or take, your dish is ready. Simply strain well, season and serve. Voila!

Here is a list of vegetables that are best served boiled. Take note of preparation times in parentheses.

spinach (1 min)
beet greens (2 min)
bean sprouts, mung or soy (2 min)
Swiss chard (3 min)

For lunch one day, try boiling a bag of bean sprouts (4 cups) and a bag of baby spinach (16 cups). This takes only 2 minutes. Lightly season with lemon and salt and prepare to be delighted by the exquisite flavor and wowed by the nutrition: 27 percent protein, 16 grams of fiber and 3 cups of water, not to mention 100 percent or more of the daily value of 6 nutrients, at just over 200 calories.

STEAMING

Steaming vegetables is an excellent way to enhance their flavor and nutrition. Steamed vegetables require very little seasoning and even less cleanup.

Steaming involves three steps. First, fill the bottom of your pot with 2 inches of water and bring it to a rapid boil. Then add vegetables to the steamer and cover. Finally, steam for the recommended time. Can it possibly get any easier?

Here are the steaming vegetables and their times.

beets (15 min)
broccoli (5 min)
Brussels sprouts (5 min)
carrots (5 min)
green cabbage (5 min)
collard greens (5 min)
green beans (5 min)
kale (5 min)
sweet potatoes (10 min)

Note how many steamed vegetables require 5 minutes to prepare. To save time and cleanup, throw several of these vegetables into the pot at once. Broccoli and kale go great together. In fact, we eat this combination almost every night! Add carrots for color. A little lemon and hot sauce and you have yourself a perfect meal!

SAUTÉING

Sautéing in broth is a superb method of preparing many different vegetables. It combines the benefits of other cooking methods into a mixture that is uniquely its own. Like stir frying, sautéing vegetables brings out their robust flavors, but without the high temperatures or oils. Like steaming, it uses moisture to soften the plant fibers and maximize nutritional benefits, provided of course that **no oil is used.** Never cook with oil. Oil is a source of empty calories. It is pure fat and devoid of nutrients, water and fiber. Moreover, heated oils can form free radicals and toxic compounds including polycyclic aromatic hydrocarbons, which terrorize your cells and accelerate aging. If you must use oil, it is better to add it to the finished dish; it is best, however, to **avoid oil altogether.** Two measly tbsp of oil have as much fat as 1 whole avocado, or 70 medium black olives! It makes sense to fulfill your fat cravings with these whole foods instead. Don't ya think?

The sauté involves three easy steps. First, heat about one inch of vegetable broth in a stainless steel skillet. The healthiest vegetable broth is made up of three components: liquid, salt and spices. Here are examples of each.

liquid: water, wine, diced tomatoes, vinegar
salt: potassium salt, Bragg's Liquid Aminos, Tabasco sauce
spices: turmeric, black pepper, dried herbs, etc.

Next, when the broth begins to steam, add your vegetables. Finally, cover and periodically stir for the recommended amount of time.

Here is a list of the vegetables that are best served sautéed, with preparation times in parentheses.

asparagus (5 min)
bell peppers (7 min)
bok choy (4 min)
red cabbage (5 min)
cauliflower (5 min)
celery (5 min)
crimini mushrooms (7 min)
eggplant (7 min)
fennel (5 min)
green peas (3 min)
garlic (1 min)
leeks (7 min)
mustard greens (3 min)
onions (7 min)
shitake mushrooms (7 min)

tomatoes (5 min)
zucchini (3 minutes)

RAW

Of course, let's not forget the easiest and possibly the healthiest method of preparing many vegetables. Raw, or *as is*.

asparagus
avocado
beets
bell peppers
broccoli
carrots
(red) cabbage
cauliflower
celery
cucumbers
fennel
green peas
garlic
herbs (basil, cilantro, dill, parsley)
kale
leeks
lettuce
mushrooms
mustard greens
olives
onions (sweet)
sea vegetables
(baby) spinach
tomatoes
zucchini

SOME ADDITIONAL TIPS

To explore different vegetables and flavors and derive a full spectrum of health benefits, *each week make use of all three forms of cooking.*

Combine 2 or more vegetables that share preparation methods. For example, steam potatoes for 5 minutes, then add kale and steam an additional 5 minutes. This saves time and cleanup.

Allow steamed vegetables (broccoli, green beans) to cool and add them to a raw salad.

To make a dish *green*, mix in some fresh baby spinach, or top with fresh herbs (basil, cilantro, dill).

Raw veggies bring cooked dishes to life. Add fresh tomatoes, onions and peppers to sautéed zucchini or asparagus and dazzle your taste buds.

To make a main course, mix in a can of beans with your vegetables, add some olive and sprinkle with yeast.

Be sure to start your dinner with a large salad or an assortment of sliced vegetable fruits (tomato, bell pepper, cucumber). This assures that your stomach is partly filled with nutritious, low calorie food before the real meal even begins.

When you crave meat, have some beans. If you desire cheese, be liberal with yeast and modest in your use of tofu. Instead of nuts or oils, have avocados or olives, and perhaps a couple tbsp of chia or flax seeds. These substitutions share the same taste receptors and eliminate cravings.

Experiment with a variety of beans. No two are alike. Chickpeas are nutty and buttery, while soybeans and kidney beans are savory. Black beans are an excellent accompaniment to spicier dishes. Mashed pinto beans mixed with onion, tomato and avocado make the perfect dip.

Also, try to satisfy all 6 taste buds each day.

> sweet: most fruits
> sour: lemon, grape, orange
> salty: potassium salt
> bitter: olives, cocoa
> savory (Umami): seaweed, mushroom, soybeans, tomatoes, carrots, yeast, soy sauce
> fat: avocado, olive, tofu, coconut milk

SOME FUN DISHES

Beans and (leafy) greens
> Boil three cups of spinach. Strain.
> Add one can of diced tomatoes or 3 whole tomatoes.
> Mix in one can of black beans.
> Sprinkle with yeast and seasonings.

Greens and beans
> Steam 3 cups broccoli and let cool.
> Add a can of kidney beans.
> Top with sliced avocado and cherry tomatoes. Spritz with lemon and sprinkle with salt.

Taste of India
> Sauté a diced red onion for 2 minutes.
> Add the florets of one whole cauliflower.
> Sauté an additional 5 minutes.
> Stir in a can of garbanzo beans.
> Add whole or canned tomatoes.
> Mix in a cup of fresh spinach.
> Strain.
> Season with turmeric until golden. Add fresh garlic and chili flakes for zest.

Spicy eggplant
> Sauté red and yellow bell peppers, onions, eggplant and crimini mushrooms for 7 minutes.
> Add diced tofu if desired.[82]
> Sprinkle with a few leaves of baby spinach.
> Season to taste.

Dip to Die For
> Sauté 1 eggplant and one 14-oz package of crimini mushrooms for 7 minutes.
> Strain and allow to cool.
> Add garlic, onion, avocado and one can of black beans.
> Puree on high in a food processor or Vita-mix blender until smooth.
> Enjoy with raw vegetables, or add it to this:

Vegetable wrap

In a large leaf of iceberg lettuce, insert one sheet of Nori seaweed.

Add the cooked vegetables of your choice. Last night's leftovers work just as well.

Top with dip, roll up and enjoy. Delicious, and perfect for lunch.

*   *   *

Of course, any green vegetable on its own makes a great main course. Diced tomatoes and garlic are the perfect accompaniment to broccoli, Brussels sprouts, green beans or leafy greens. A can of beans provides additional flavor and savor.

One cooked green atop one raw leafy green, mixed with 1 vegetable fruit and 1 fatty fruit make the perfect meal and could easily be consumed daily. For example, lay steamed broccoli on a bed of lettuce with sliced tomato and ½ an avocado.

Dijon mustard, yeast, lemon and Tabasco mixed together makes the perfect dressing.

Make a meal of mushrooms. Buy a 24-oz package of white or brown mushrooms, rinse well, slice into quarters and season with salt, yeast flakes and cayenne pepper. Then, turn on your favorite movie and enjoy as you would popcorn. It's only 150 calories, compared to over 500 calories in microwave popcorn.

If you are still unsure how to fit fruits and vegetables into your daily life at every meal, this may help.

A DAY IN YOUR LIFE

<u>Breakfast</u>
As fruit is best consumed alone, it is most convenient to enjoy it first and foremost: that is, in a fruit salad, as individual whole fruits or preferably blended in a shake.

Once again, here are the essentials of a fruit shake:
Juicy fruit (melon, citrus)
Concentrated fruit (banana, dates, avocado, prunes)
Antioxidant fruit (berries)
Leafy green (optional)

If eating fruit and only fruit for breakfast is the only change you make to your diet, you will reap significant health benefits, including weight loss and increased vitality.

The cleansing affect of fruit greatly enhances the digestive process, and the quick energy its simple sugars provide promises to reduce cravings later in the day.

Indeed it is wiser to skip your morning meal altogether than to eat what is commonly served at most breakfast tables (animal foods and processed grains). Most commercial cereals, and almost all breads, muffins, bagels and pastries are high glycemic, nutrient-starved foods that give a brief burst of energy followed by hours of fatigue and food cravings. Thanks a lot! Animal products (meat, cheese, eggs and milk) feature so prominently at breakfast time that one wonders how anybody can face the day with such a heavy load in her stomach. And what is worse, these concentrated foods are often combined, which by now you know spells disaster. Even a body-builder's breakfast of oatmeal and egg whites - which by the standards of most seems pretty healthy, as it is high in protein and low in fat - is actually quite lacking, especially in carbohydrates (brain food), fiber and many major nutrients.

<u>1 cup cooked oatmeal, 6 egg whites</u>

400 calories
56 g carbohydrates
32.5 g protein
6 g fat
7.5 g fiber
vitamin A 0

vitamin C 0
calcium: 5
iron: 48
25% or more DV of 8 nutrients

vs.

<u>2 bananas,5 prunes, 6 tbsp nutritional yeast</u>

480 calories
109 g carbohydrates
21.5 g protein
3 g fat
19 g fiber
13 vitamin A
34 vitamin C
3 calcium
33 iron
25% or more DV of 13 nutrients

Look at that nutrition, we say!
Yuck, you may reply.

This is, of course, just an example to show the protein and fiber contributions of yeast. It is preferred to mix yeast with vegetables rather than to have it with fruit for breakfast, so please do not attempt that recipe at home. We did once. Got through it, but it wasn't pretty.

Speaking of breakfast, do you really need it, as nutritionists claim? Is breakfast the most important meal of the day? Well, yes and no.

If you eat a nutritious dinner the night before, or just by eating a sufficient number of calories, your body is able to store 200 grams (800 calories) of glucose, enough energy for ten to eighteen hours of fasting.

In other words, if you ate dinner last night at 8 PM, then you have sufficient fuel packed in your liver to get you to at least lunch, even if you exercise in the morning. You see, muscle has a storage pool of an additional 300 grams or 1,200 calories of glucose, which would last you for a 12-mile long run. (*Who the heck runs 12 miles before breakfast?!* we hear you scream. One day, you will.) And when your stored glucose runs dry your liver can manufacture it from last night's dietary proteins and fats. This process is known as *gluconeogenesis*. Literally, making new sugar.

In short, unless you skip dinner the night before or plan to run a marathon, you don't even need breakfast. Your body has enough fuel on which to function.

This is why it is **better** to skip breakfast rather than load up on refined grains and animal products, which serve only to weigh your digestion down. Of course nutritious breakfasts bring with them a lot of perks: A healthy morning meal encourages improved attention, quicker and more accurate retrieval of information, fewer mistakes and better concentration and ability to perform complex tasks. In other words, you are more likely to make an A, or get a raise, if you *eat well in the AM*.

And so...

As far as breakfast is concerned, it is **best** to eat fruit and fruit alone. Fruit is a source of rapidly-digested energy that does not bring with it the lows that come with high glycemic foods such as most breakfast cereals. It contains more carbohydrate than meat and dairy, which have little if any energy. And by now you know that plant food is the most nutritious stuff on Earth.

Eating fruit in the AM is like taking a water and fiber-packed multivitamin, with added energy. And the sweetness goes straight to the brain. Brain fuel, remember? Glucose is after all the brain's preferred energy source. So choose fruit.

You could eat vegetables, but most vegetables are high in protein and starch relative to fruit and therefore require more digestive effort. Vegetables are therefore best consumed at your evening meal.

For breakfast, choose fruit.

If a few pieces of sweet juicy fruit does not satisfy you, or if you feel you require more calories, include concentrated fruits such as bananas and dates. Or mix in some dried fruits (prunes, figs, raisins). Aim for a combination of at least 5 whole fruits and 3 cups of fruits each and every day, more if you are active.

Since quantity is the goal, when consuming whole fruits, start with juicy fruit, which is more nutritious and less caloric. Then, move to concentrated fruits. Or better yet, blend them all together in a refreshing smoothie.

<u>Dinner</u>

The perfect dinner consists of three courses.

1. A large salad or several pieces of raw vegetables (bell peppers, cucumber, carrots, mushrooms, tomatoes)
2. A lightly cooked green vegetable dish
3. Beans and/or potatoes, or a second vegetable dish

The large salad should be a major feature of dinner. Simply grab a bowl and fill with as much leafy greens, vegetable fruits and fatty fruits as you like. In fact, let your eyes be bigger than your stomach. Chances are that your stomach has shrunk due to a lifetime of small portions of calorically dense processed grains and animal products. Your stomach is actually quite larger than you think. In fact, an empty stomach has a volume of 1.5 L and a capacity of 3 L or more! That's 12 glasses of water![83] To get a visual of this, find a 3 L Tupperware container and fill it with vegetables. This is how much your stomach can accommodate, *at least*. As with anything of value - running faster, getting stronger, earning better grades, making the world a better place - improvement takes practice. You have to learn to eat larger and larger meals in order to expand your stomach and accustom it to greater bulk. But remember, the bulk is just the packaging, designed by nature to deliver the nutrients to your cells and help your system eliminate waste. If you shrank 3 L of fruits and veggies down by removing the water and fiber, you'd be left with about 5 percent volume, or 1.25 oz. If that volume were alcohol, it wouldn't even be enough to get you drunk, let alone make you fat.

And once you get the hang of eating water and fiber-rich foods, you won't settle for anything less. The small, saturated stuff filled with fat and drenched in chemicals just won't suit you any more. Your taste buds will have reverted to their natural state. They no longer will be tantalized by rich sauces, heavy fats and syrupy glazes. Rather, they will crave freshness and crunchiness, clean wholesome food that is lip-smacking good.

So for your salad, fill the bowl (or Tupperware) with lettuce, the darker the leaf the better. Romaine, red leaf or arugula will do, and feel free to mix in some baby spinach. Then, add diced cucumbers, tomatoes, bell peppers and perhaps some onions. Finally, top with olives and avocado. Spritz in some lemon and add a shake or two of sea salt. Don't be intimidated by the quantity. Remember, these foods are mostly (85 percent or more) water, and much of what remains is fiber. Both are calorie-free and filling. Your stomach is able to quickly and easily absorb the water in fruits and vegetables, which decreases the sensation of fullness that would endure for a painfully long period if you were to eat a large quantity of concentrated food (animal products, grains, nuts). So eat a huge bowl of plants. You won't feel stuffed, trust us!

Then, lightly cook one or two of your favorite vegetables and have this as the perfect companion to raw vegetables, either atop the salad or as the main course. If you require or desire additional calories, add beans. For added flavor and nutrition, top with nutritional yeast and make appropriate use of other condiments.

We can hear you wondering: *Fruit for breakfast and lunch followed by a three-course dinner? I thought you're not supposed to eat big meals before bed!*

Glad you're thinking. The whole *eat like a king for breakfast, a prince for lunch and a pauper at supper* philosophy is another myth to dispel. Look at it this way. Digestion uses up a ton of energy (thermic effect of food, requiring 10 percent or more of your day's calories, remember?). This energy is better devoted to other activities (exercise, school, work, etc.). It makes sense that the food you consume during the day be light and rapidly absorbed with little digestive effort, which as we know is fruit. Then you can save yourself for a big evening feast, after which you can tuck yourself into bed and allow your body to devote its energies fully to digesting and absorbing those nutrients.

Do you doubt?

To better understand this, let's learn a thing or two about how your nervous system works.

Your nervous system is divided into two parts, central and peripheral. Your central nervous system consists of your brain and spinal cord. Your peripheral nervous system leaves your brain and spinal cord and travels out to your body. It is further divided into two parts: voluntary and involuntary. The voluntary (somatic) nervous system is under your conscious control. It is what gets activated when you flex a muscle or pucker up to kiss your loved one. (Well, the involuntary nervous system may get activated too, sending "butterflies" through your stomach). The involuntary nervous system is also called the autonomic nervous system (autonomic like automatic, as in not under your control). In contrast to the voluntary system, which moves your muscles, the autonomic system governs the functions of your organs (heart, lungs, intestines, etc.).

Don't get lost in the details. This is just background information. The involuntary/autonomic nervous system is further divided into sympathetic and parasympathetic arms.

NERVOUS SYSTEM

Central   Peripheral
           Somatic----Autonomic
           Sympathetic------Parasympathetic

The sympathetic nervous system is active in *fight or flight* responses. It gets turned on in times of stress, such as when you face a challenge and need to decide whether to attack it or run the other way. This may be a bully in the playground or a new job prospect. Whatever your choice, the sympathetic nervous system fills your lungs with air and pumps your muscles full of blood. It says *focus* and *act* and uses neurotransmitters such as adrenaline – hence, the *adrenaline rush* that comes when you are excited, scared or working towards a deadline. By contrast, the parasympathetic nervous system is your body's housekeeper. Its domain is *rest and digest*. The acronym taught in medical school is SLUDGE, which stands for salivation, lacrimation, urination, defecation, gastrointestinal processes and emesis, another word for vomiting. All of these are related to food, and food is under the control of the parasympathetic.

Sympathetic
"fight and flight"

Parasympathetic
"rest and digest"

Are you catching on? Yes, these two systems oppose each other. Well, oppose is a bit harsh. Let's say that they complement each other - with opposite actions. For one to function best, the other needs to be dormant. When one turns on, the other turns off. (For example, the parasympathetic nervous system controls erection, while the sympathetic nervous system causes ejaculation.) Which is why, when you feel stressed out, you may get a stomachache or feel constipated. The sympathetic nervous system shuts down your digestion and moves blood to your brain, heart and muscles until the stressor has been dealt with, at which time the parasympathetic can once again move contents through your bowels. Maybe you have been told not to swim after eating. The principle is the same: Activate the sympathetic nervous system with muscle activity, and the parasympathetic nervous system shuts off, food is inadequately digested and vomiting can ensue. If your body digests the meal rather than provide exercising muscles with blood, what you get are cramps as a result of lactic acid build-up (courtesy of anaerobic respiration) and the consequent danger of drowning. So listen to your mother and don't swim on a full belly.

At this point, let's ask ourselves a question. If the sympathetic nervous system helps you meet deadlines and face challenges, and the parasympathetic is active when you rest and digest, does it not make sense then to let the parasympathetic system work unopposed and to rest and digest simultaneously? This is what you allow to happen when you go to bed on a full stomach. You sleep (rest) and digest, quiet, still and stress free, letting your sympathetic nervous system sleep with you while the parasympathetic arm assimilates your food. In the morning you awake with a full tank, ready to greet the day.

If in the past you have suffered restless sleep or unpleasant dreams after consuming a big meal before bed, try and recall exactly what it was you ate. Chances are it was heavy food featuring some combination of breads, pasta, meat and sauces, cheese, pies, oils and butter. These foods will upset your system at any time of the day, any season of the year. This won't happen with fruits and vegetables. If you don't trust us, conduct an experiment of your own, for as they say: Life is an experiment of one. This means YOU!

<u>Dessert</u>

If you crave sweets after dinner, a piece of whole fruit or a few slices of melon is often all that you need. If you require more than this, you may not have consumed enough food for dinner. If like some you prefer to derive more calories from dessert than from dinner, a frozen banana mixed with a few dates or figs is concentrated, satisfying and delicious - and best enjoyed after raw rather than cooked vegetables.

Lunch

We left lunch for last for a reason.

Incorporating the Paradigm Diet at your lunchtime meal is likely the biggest challenge you'll face. If you are like most, you eat lunch outside the home (at work or school), which means that if you pack a lunch, it has to be pre-made. Unlike some meat dishes, vegetable leftovers retain their flavor and nutrition for several days, if covered and refrigerated. If you are willing to prepare your or your loved one's lunch, invest in large (2 L) Tupperware containers with airtight sealing capability, preferably the type that snaps closed.

Here are a few lunchtime suggestions:

Mix last night's leftover vegetables over a large bed of lettuce. The lettuce will awaken them. For additional flavor, spritz with lemon and add tapenade and Tabasco.

Include 1-2 pieces of fruit and have them a few minutes before your meal.

A lunch exclusively of fruit is also an option, and one we abide by every day, weekends and holidays included. Why? Because we love it! Fruit is easy to buy, easy to eat, sweet, tasty and nourishing. Lunch trucks, corner stores and gas stations even carry fruit. To reduce quantity and make carrying it easier, include concentrated fruit for lunch, such as bananas and dates. (More than once, we've made a luncheon feast of exclusively bananas, eating six at a sitting. We would have preferred a bag of oranges, but nothing else was available.) If you can store your food in a refrigerator, pack a fruit salad. Diced fruit is best eaten the same day, but it can last up to a week. Try adding Romaine lettuce or other vegetables to your fruit salad, include a touch of salt, and prepare to be delighted by the sweet and salty sensation.

Another option is to steam 100 calories worth of a vegetable (broccoli), mix in diced tomatoes and 1 can of beans (rinsed and strained). Season to taste. You can make enough to last a few days, if you wish, as I did in medical school and in residency. This lunch takes 5 minutes to make and is practically cleanup free. And it really packs a punch.

Punch-packing Lunch
2 cups steamed broccoli: 90 calories, 10 g fiber
1.5 cups kidney beans: 325 calories, 25 g fiber
1 cup diced tomatoes: 100 calories, 4 g fiber

Nutritional value
515 calories
75-20-5
39 grams fiber
at least 25% of the DV of 16 essential nutrients

You may find as you increase your consumption of Paradigm foods that it is best to reserve old habits (pizza, chips, sandwiches) for lunchtime, while eating fruit for breakfast and for dessert, and eating exclusively vegetables for dinner. Lunch habits, especially if they include sandwiches, are usually last to go. Old habits die hard, as they say. And while we recognize that for many people sandwiches are easy and satisfying, we must remind you that **so is fruit.**

Let's compare a peanut butter and jelly sandwich to a mix of bananas and dates:

Peanut butter and jelly sandwich
2 slices whole wheat bread
2 heaping tbsp peanut butter
2 tbsp jelly
610 calories
fat: 34 grams
fiber: 7 grams

vs.

2 bananas, 6 dates
609 calories
fat: 1 gram
fiber: 16 grams

And remember that both iceberg lettuce and sheets of Nori seaweed make great alternatives to bread and tortilla, as do collard greens. Wrap last night's vegetables into these leafy greens for a much more nutritious version of the standard wrap.

If you get a chance to *eat in* for lunch, let us interest you in the lunchtime smoothie. It is like the breakfast shake, only a bit more vegetable-centric and hearty, to satisfy you till dinner.

Green Smoothie
enough for 2 people
1 package (10 oz) baby spinach
½ cup water
2 tbsp flax seed
2 tbsp cocoa powder
2 tbsp cinnamon
2 frozen (or fresh) bananas
1 cup fresh (or frozen) strawberries
stevia (no-calorie herbal sweetener) to taste
<u>Directions:</u>
Blend the baby spinach with water until it liquefies.
Add the cocoa powder, cinnamon and flax seed.
Mix in the bananas and strawberries and blend until smooth.
Sprinkle in some stevia for added sweetness, if desired.

This smoothie makes 4 cups, and you and a friend can have 2 cups each. The flax seed is high in omega-3 fatty acids. The cocoa powder and cinnamon provide additional flavor and are also very high in antioxidants.

In fact, by weight, many spices contain more antioxidant capability than berries. The problem is, most of us don't consume enough cinnamon or cocoa to really glean the benefit. Although a shake here and there can please the palate, it won't do your cells much good unless you measure your spice by the tablespoonful, in which case you can easily exceed the free-radical fighting potency of even the most potent fruits and vegetables.

To illustrate: One cup of blueberries provides 6,225 ORAC units, which is less than the amount in 1 tbsp of ground cinnamon! So get out your measuring spoon. Other nutritious spices include turmeric, cayenne, sage and clove. Basil, rosemary, dill, oregano and thyme are excellent dried herbs.[84]

The lunchtime smoothie is a tasty vehicle for leafy greens, omega-3s and anti-oxidant spices to get into your system, at under 300 calories per serving. Drink at least 2 cups, and don't be intimidated by quantity. Since your stomach can hold 12 cups of liquid, you can handle 2 or 3 cups or more, no problem.

IN SUMMARY
(just in case you need a little reinforcement)

<u>Fruit for breakfast</u>
A big (4 cup) shake with sweet juicy fruit (melon, citrus), high ORAC fruit (berries), concentrated fruit (banana), provides at least 6 of your target 8 daily servings of fruits. Greens (spinach) and seeds (chia, flax) are optional, as are spices (cocoa, cayenne, cinnamon).

<u>Mid-morning snack</u>
1 or 2 fresh fruits, either whole or as part of a fruit salad. Have more if desired.

<u>Lunch and Dinner</u>
Any combination that taken together equals:
- 1 lb cooked vegetables (broccoli, cauliflower, kale)
- 1 lb raw vegetables and vegetable fruits (mushrooms, bell peppers, cucumbers)
- 1 or 2 fatty fruits (avocado, olives)
- 2 or 3 servings of legumes (beans, peas, lentils)
- 2 or 3 servings of starches (potatoes, sweet potatoes, carrots, squash)

<u>Dessert</u>
Fresh fruit, if desired.

Together these foods fulfill the recommended intake of most vitamins and minerals, can be purchased for around $100 per week, require cooking times of under 10 minutes and preparation times (including chopping and cleaning up) of less than 30 minutes.

Making the Paradigm Diet part of your life is so easy, you may wish to begin right now.

"Let's Get Started" Salad
(serves 1 or 2)
1 head of Romaine lettuce
½ avocado
¼ diced red onion
1 tomato
1 cucumber
1 lemon (juice)
1 can black beans
1 tbsp Dijon
1 tbsp Tabasco
2 tbsp yeast
salt to taste

Preparation: Chop the vegetables. Add the beans. Mix in the condiments. Enjoy.

COURSE FOUR: PARADIGM FITNESS

Ever asked yourself what makes us human? You know, what makes you YOU?

So as not to drown ourselves in philosophical debate, let's keep it simple.

There's your body, which we've been discussing this whole time. Then there is your mind, for as Descartes said, "I think therefore I am." Everything else let's just call your spirit or soul, which also makes you who you are, even though you cannot see it. We're pyramids, each of us: bodies, minds and souls. And the body - what we put into it and what we do with it - is the base.

Like twin pillars, **fitness** and **nutrition** are the foundation on which reside the other components of a healthy life. These include loving relationships, service to others, artistic expression, recreational pursuits and problem solving.

Without adequate nourishment and sufficient physical activity, living a full and fulfilling life is like building a castle in the clouds: It admits no prospect of success.

As with nutrition, a scientific approach can be applied to the realm of physical fitness. First we must ask, what are the elements of physical fitness? Reasoning scientifically, the name itself suggests our answer.

The descriptive term *physical* pertains to the body, specifically its *composition* (body weight and body mass distribution, also known as body fat percentage), and its *activity* level, as concerns strength, stamina and flexibility, or stretching.

Fitness implies the extent to which the body is able to engage in a given activity. Fitness, or performance, is a function of one's physicality. In general, the more superb your body's composition and the more regularly active you are, the greater your fitness.

For example, the more weights you lift, the more your muscles grow and the stronger you get. The farther and more frequently you run, the lighter you become and the greater are your efficiency and endurance. And only through regular stretching are you able to perform the splits, which we are unable to do. Oh, well. Guess we'll have to just keep on stretching!

Here then are the three components of physical fitness:

PHYSICAL
1. Body composition
body weight
body fat percentage

2. Activity level(exercise)
strength
stamina
stretching

FITNESS
3. Maximum activity

As maximum activity (fitness) is a function of body composition and activity level (physicality), we can maximize fitness by achieving our ideal body composition and engaging in the optimal amount of exercise.

Let's take a moment to explore in depth the 3 components of physical fitness.

BODY COMPOSITION

Body composition is a function of two things: your body weight and your body fat percentage.

Body weight

How much do you weigh? How much should you weigh? For our answer we turn to what's known as body mass index, or BMI.

BMI is a two-digit number derived from the ratio of your weight to your height. Specifically, it is your weight in lbs x 703, divided by your height, in inches squared. Or if you prefer the metric system, your weight in kg divided by your height, in meters squared. If you don't fancy these formulas, tables and Internet calculators make figuring your BMI quick and easy.[85]

How important is the BMI? Doctors use it to determine your health risks, and life insurance companies go by it when calculating liability, which determines your monthly premium. Depending on your BMI value, you are considered underweight, normal, overweight or obese.

Normal: Between 18.5 and 24.9.

Underweight: Below 18.5.

Overweight: Between 25 and 30.

Obese: 30 or above.

How accurate a predictor of health is the BMI? Not very. As it turns out, the BMI has a few flaws.

First, as muscle is denser than fat, a very muscular person can be classified as overweight/unhealthy when he is anything but.

Also, the BMI is not gender-specific. Healthy weights are the same regardless of your sex, which allows for misinterpretation and inaccuracies, as we'll explore in a jiff.

Next, BMI tables allow for ranges that are ludicrously wide. For example, a healthy weight for a 5'10" person is anywhere between 132 and 174 lbs. That's a range of over 40 lbs!

To put this in perspective: Let's say you weigh 135 lbs (BMI: 19) and your friend weighs 170 (BMI 24). You are the same height and have similar muscle mass. Is your friend, who carries an additional 35 lbs of fat, as healthy as you?

Um, no.

If you need proof, offer to race said friend. The extra weight she carries is like having a 20 lb ankle weight attached to each leg. You're sure to be more swift-footed, even if you are less conditioned, as an elegant study conducted at Yale comparing the athletic performance of vegetarians and meat-eaters showed.[86]

In truth, health problems appear at BMIs of 22 and up. Yet according to the standard that health professionals use, your friend is as healthy as you. Hey, that's not fair!

BMI is calculated the same way for kids (ages 2 to 20) as for adults, but its interpretation differs slightly. Kids are assigned a percentile based on their body mass index, which factors in changes in body fat percentage that occur with age. A healthy weight is between the 5th and 85th percentiles. This is from 120 lbs (BMI of 17) to 165 lbs (BMI of 24.5) for a 5'10", 16-year-old boy or girl. Again, a huge range.

We are not saying that everyone of a given height should weigh exactly the same. Like snowflakes, no 2 people are exactly alike, not even identical twins. Individual variations do exist. They are attributable to differences in gender and in frame size. Generally, men weigh more than women. Also, small-framed people weigh less than medium-sized people, who tend to be lighter than big-framed folks.

To determine your frame size, wrap your left hand around your right wrist, at the crease where your arm meets your palm. Try to touch your left middle finger with your left thumb. If you cannot, you are large framed. If your fingers barely touch, you are of medium build. If they overlap, you are small-framed.[87]

So, if BMI is an unreliable predictor of health, how do you know how much you should weigh? As it turns out, the BMI is not totally useless. As mentioned, weight-associated health problems begin to appear at BMIs of 22,[88] so for starters it's best to be below this. The following gender-specific formulas put you at the lighter half of *normal* (BMI 17 to 21), which is the true healthy range.

If you are a female: Take **95** lbs for the first 5 feet of height and add or subtract **4** lbs for every inch above or below.

For example:

4'10"	95 − 8 = 87 lbs (BMI 18)
5'0"	95 + 0 = 95 lbs (BMI 19)
5'4"	95 + 16 = 111 lbs (BMI 19)
5'8"	95 + 32 = 127 lbs (BMI 19)
5'10"	95 + 40 = 135 lbs (BMI 19)

If you are a male: Start with **100** lbs for the first 5 feet of height and add/subtract **5** lbs for every inch above/below. A 5'10" male should weigh approximately 150 lbs (BMI 21.5). Medium-framed and larger-framed individuals may add 5 or 10 lbs to their ideal weight, to take into account heavier skeletons and denser musculature.

Today's date:
My current body weight:
My ideal body weight:

Wait a minute! we hear you saying. *These weights seem awfully low to me. I consider myself normal and you're telling me I need to lose 20 lbs??? F(*&%, man, you're giving me a complex!*

We hear you, and the intention is not to wound your self esteem. But the truth is, by comparison to the roughly 2 in 3 people that are overweight, and the 1 in 3 that are obese (severely overweight), carrying a little extra body fat, maybe even a lot of extra body fat, seems normal. But with so much sickness and disease, normal no longer means healthy. So, fix your diet and the weight will naturally melt away, this we promise!

If you are still not convinced of your ideal body weight, and still harboring resentment at the audacity that possessed us to suggest such a freakin' low weight as normal, we have a solution, if a temporary one.

Think back to your childhood. Recall the moment in the past when you reached your adult height. Early bloomers like us may have topped out at the age of 14 or 15, while others grow taller through college. Try and remember what you weighed way back when. Chances are as a teen you were more active than now, so your weight when you achieved your adult height can be considered a set point, at least for the time being. (In other words, until you get even leaner!)

<u>Body fat percentage</u>

As the name implies, your body fat percentage indicates how much of your body mass is made up of fat. The remainder, or whatever is not fat, is referred to as lean body mass.

Lean body mass = Total body weight - Body fat

It is universally accepted that due to differences in body composition (for example, breasts and hips) women generally have more body fat than men. However, opinions vary about what constitutes the right amount of fat. What is the ideal percentage of body fat for either sex?

The American Council on Exercise uses the following classifications:[89]

	Women	Men
Essential fat	10-12%	2-4%
Athletes	14-20%	6-13%
Fitness	21-24%	14-17%
Acceptable	25-31%	18-25%
Obese	32% or more	26% or more

This is conventional, but is it wisdom?

Fat cells serve a very limited function. It is true that they manufacture hormones such as estrogen, but the ovaries and adrenals also produce estrogen. Fat provides insulation, but this function has become largely outdated and replaced by warm clothing, heaters (and global warming, you might add). Mainly, fat cells serve as a storage site for fats (energy) and toxins (waste).

In famine, body fat is our best defense against starvation. In fact, your fat cells provide enough fuel (135,000 calories) for over 2 months in the absence of food. But do you plan to starve? No. In the modern era of abundance, famine is largely extinct. (Although, the modern diet of fast food does induce a sort of nutrient starvation, and the environmental effects of factory farming make future famine a possibility.) Is it appropriate then, that a body fat percentage in excess of 25 percent of one's weight be considered acceptable? Unless you're planning on hibernating for the winter, the answer is clearly NO.

For ideal body fat percentage, we must turn to more conservative estimates.[90]

	Women	Men
FIT	**13-19%**	**3-9%**
Full-bodied	20-24%	10-14%
Fat	25%+	15%+

As far as fat is concerned, it is wise to be conservative. Ignore the two bottom rows and concentrate on the first: **Body fat in the single digits for men, and in the teens for women, should be regarded as ideal.** Kids generally have more body fat than adults, so higher values may apply.

Of the two – body weight and body fat – body fat is indicative of greater fitness. Why? It's intuitive, really. Less fat means more lean muscle mass, and muscle is more metabolically active. Our muscles are responsible for movement. They rapidly burn ATP to pump blood through the circulation, push food through the GI tract and propel our bodies in motion. Active cells make for active bodies. Fat cells, which are relatively inert, require fewer calories.

How to calculate your body fat? As with body weight, useful and accurate formulas exist.

First, to determine your weight, step on an accurate scale. It is best to do this naked, in the morning, *before* breakfast and *after* a bowel movement. To verify the accuracy of your scale, lay upon it a 5-lb dumbbell or other object of known mass.

Once you determine your weight, take the following measurements:

1. waist at the navel (belly button): _____
2. hips at their widest point: _____

3. neck: _____
4. height (without shoes): _____

Finally, go to any one among a number of useful websites, such as livestrong.com or healthstatus.com, input your measurements and determine your body fat percentage. Then, compare it to the values above, to see how you measure up.

Today's date: _____
My body fat percentage: _____

* * *

In terms of health, what is more important, body weight or body fat percentage? Simple. It is better to be overweight but with an ideal amount of body fat, than to weigh the perfect amount but carry excessive blubber. Visceral fat, the kind which covers your vital organs, especially in your abdomen, and which may not be noticeable in thinner individuals, is associated with cancer, heart disease and diabetes. Its cause? We bet you can answer this question yourself by now: saturated fat and trans fats, of course, as occur in animal foods and processed grains.

Yet, even muscular people should avoid gaining too much weight. An *obese* bodybuilder - pardon the oxymoron, in other words a densely muscularized, very heavy individual of little body fat such as you might see posing in bikini trunks on the Mr. Olympia dais, or in any of the *Conan* movies - requires a strong heart capable of supplying blood to all that extra mass; and as muscle is more active than fat, the heart of a 300-lb bodybuilder must be much stronger, for it must work much harder, than the heart of a 300-lb flabby person. In order to strengthen the heart, the bodybuilder had best engage in strenuous heart-pumping cardiovascular activity, which weightlifters sometimes shun, for fear of losing muscle mass.

And so, *it is best to be both low in body fat and on or around your ideal body weight.* In other words, it is best to be **lean**. Being lean (light weight, low body fat) conduces to extensive physical activity, since muscles are the most active; and only through extensive activity can you become lean. So the two go together.

Really, though, there is no reason to be a slave to your weight. Weight is just a number, and rather than obsess, you can forget about the lbs. Once you eat the right foods, your body will recalibrate. Fewer toxins in, means less of a need for storage sites (fat), resulting in weight loss. In addition, good clean food will improve your mood, your muscles and movement will increase and the rest will follow effortlessly.

ACTIVITY LEVEL

Having defined your ideal body weight and body fat percentage, we can next turn our attention to the recommended amount of activity in the three areas of fitness: strength, stamina and stretching.

Exercise is defined as *bodily exertion for the sole sake of training and the benefits of health.* This definition neglects the highest purpose of exercise, and this is *to just plain have fun.*

In grade school, daily time is allotted for play. For 15 minutes at ten AM and maybe thirty minutes at lunch, you got to horse around, yell and scream, hide and seek, goof off, just be a kid. You got to exercise. In fact, you were (or are) forced to exercise, but because it is fun, it doesn't seem forced at all.[91] A more focused if less fun approach to exercise continues in high school with PE (physical education) and organized sports for the talented and driven.[92]

Once you graduate high school, if you aren't a member of a sports team, the choice to continue being active is up to you. And just as some choose not to enroll in college, many teens opt out of exercising.[93]

The average weight gain in the first 12 weeks of freshman year of college is almost 5 lbs. It's called *the freshman five.*[94] Kept up, that's nearly 20 lbs per year. And it gets worse after college, as metabolism can slow with age. If as you grow older you become less active, your muscle mass decreases and your metabolism slackens to the same degree.[95]

With time, bad habits multiply like weeds and become very difficult to uproot. Thus the saying: *You can't teach an old dog new tricks.* As they grow older, people become as inactive as potted plants, and married to their dietary indiscretions. (How many times have you heard a person say, *I love my cheese,* as though it belonged to her alone. If you are such a person and you have cellulite, your cheese not only belongs to you, it *is* you.)

Staying active involves the conscious decision to do so. Giving yourself the option to work out if you feel like it often leads to taking a nap, watching TV, eating a snack – or possibly doing all three!

It is therefore wise to familiarize yourself with the recommended activities and do them on most days of the week, at least, or better yet make exercise part of your daily routine. Just as you *take time* to brush your teeth, watch TV, kiss your sweetheart, visit the toilet and drink coffee or tea, so should you *make time* to move around. Exercise has a dose response effect, meaning more is better.

The American College of Sports Medicine and the American Heart Association make these minimum exercise guidelines:

Stamina
* **30 minutes, 5 times a week of moderate cardiovascular exercise** (60 percent of maximum effort);

Or:

* **20 minutes, 3 times a week of vigorous cardio** (80 percent of maximum effort);[96]

And:

Strength
* **10 sets of strength exercises, 8-12 reps each, twice weekly.**

You can estimate you percent maximum effort as follows:

1. Maximum heart rate (220 minus age in years): _____

2. Multiply #1 x .6: _____

3. Multiply #1 x .8: _____

The number you come up with in #2 is 60 percent of maximum effort. The value in #3 is 80 percent maximal effort. Between these values is your **target heart rate**.

Example: Aaron is 37.
   1. Subtracting his age from 220 yields *183*. This is his **maximum heart rate**.
   3. Multiply 183 x .6 equals *110*. This is 60 percent maximal effort.
   3. 183 x .8 equals *146*. This is 80 percent maximum effort.

For maximum cardiovascular benefit, Aaron should maintain a heart rate in the 110 to 146 beats per minute (bpm) range. This is his **target heart rate.**

If stopping and checking your heart rate each time you exercise seems like too much work, just do it once. You'll remember the level of effort associated with your heart rate values. Another way to determine your level of exertion is to use your breathing and speaking effort. If while running you can keep up a conversation with little difficulty, you are at or around the 60 percent range. If you cannot talk without gasping for breath, you are likely closer to 80 percent of your maximum heart rate. Alternatively, if while running it takes you three steps to inhale and three to exhale, you are exercising at about 60 percent effort. More rapid breathing rates correlate with greater intensity.

It's okay to take it easy some days. Lower levels of exertion (less than 50 percent of your maximum) burn more fat than higher levels of intensity, which use carbohydrate as their major source of fuel.[97] But don't use this as an excuse to slack off. Remember that for the same length of time, the faster your run, the farther you go, and the more calories you burn. The type of calorie burned is less important than the overall amount. Even if carbohydrates are your fuel, if you burn enough of them, fat loss will follow.

Also, from time to time you may wish to take your heart rate above its maximum. Periodic bursts of power or speed that reach the maximum heart rate (as in sprints or squats) are of both muscle-building and fat-burning benefit, a combination that is rarely achieved in other forms of exercise.

Whatever your level of exertion, working out should be enjoyable. So keep it fun.

Stretch

There exist no stretch (flexibility) guidelines, so we must come up with our own. Most will find it is useful to stretch after exercise or on its own, as part of your routine.

SUMMARY OF EXERCISE RECOMMENDATIONS

Stamina: a minimum of 25 minutes at 70 percent maximum effort on most (4) days of the week, on average.

Strength: 10 sets of resistance, twice weekly.

Stretch: daily.

INTRODUCTION TO EXERCISES

Stamina

Running

The champion of exercises, running is simple, effective and convenient. Anthropologists believe that the human form is a function of our ancestors' need to run. Whether running in search of food or so as not to become food, we ran. A lot. In fact, it was not uncommon for prehistoric man to run as much as 16 or 20 hours each day. Over long distances, humans can outrun the fastest animals, at times even beating the horse, as the annual Man Against Horse 50-mile race in Arizona has shown. Other evidence - that we walk on two legs, have little body hair and lots of sweat glands, in addition to a nuchal ligament and a mobile 1st vertebral joint - all points to the same thing:

We were born to run.[98]

Running is our natural state, and yet few do it enough if at all. Instead, we spend 8 hours or more each day at the desk and in the car, with additional time slouched on the couch and scarfing grub at the table. Added to the 8 hours we sleep, this amounts to 16 to 20 hours per day or more spent on our backs and backsides. Back in Nature, we used to run that much!

Now, you've probably been told not to run. Maybe you've even said it. *Running will ruin your joints*, some say. Others have remarked: *I used to run, but it broke down my back*. In fact, the opposite is true: Today's set-up is totally unnatural. The sedentary life is ruining us. Sitting at a desk is leaving us stiff and bent over. We get old because we stop running, and remain young as long as we move! Stagnant water sits still. The clear stream flows forward.

Run any place, any time. Do it indoors or outdoors, rain or shine. At the park or in the mountains, up a hill, on a track, around your block or on your treadmill. All you need is the spirit of adventure (shoes are optional, unnecessary and may even be harmful).[99] Run soft and straight. Keep your head steady and let your arms gracefully sway at your sides as your feet touch down quickly and turn over rapidly. If this seems like too much instruction, just take your shoes off and run in the grass. Perfect form will come naturally.

Riding

Another beautiful way to move, bicycling is easy on your joints and builds very muscular legs. What's more, even as a beginner you can go much faster and farther than you ever could on foot. Invest in a mountain bike if you live by a trail, or buy a road bike and hit the paths, boardwalk or well-paved road. (Used bikes start at a mere $100. Remember, it's not the bike but what you do with it that counts.)

Ride to school or to work and bookmark the day with twin workouts (you'll have to ride home at the day's end). In cold weather, invest in a resistance trainer and you have an instant stationary bike that fits in any room, yard or garage. Find a hill near you and scale it a couple times, even if you have to zig-zag your way to the top. There will come a day when you'll go straight up, like a shooting star, only in reverse.

Roping

Most have jumped rope at some point in life. And what they say about riding a bike can be said here as well. It's easy and you never really forget. Roping allows you to take your workout with you wherever you go. And unlike running or riding, your upper body gets just as much of a burn as your lower body. Buy a beaded rope for about ten dollars and get into the swing. Aim for at least 100 skips per minute. One thousand skips is equivalent to a 1-mile run.

Swimming

All this gem of an exercise requires is a pool, a suit and a pair of goggles. If you don't have a pool, the YMCA is only a car or bike ride away. Freestyle and breaststroke are two of the best and most efficient strokes. Try the butterfly if you get really experienced. Even just treading water works well.

Strength

Body weight

Before the advent of gyms, bodybuilders relied on Nature's gift to furnish them with their strength training. Exercises such as pull-ups, pushups, dips, handstand presses, body weight squats, sit-ups and leg raises provide a total body workout. They hit all of the major muscle groups - shoulders, arms, back, legs and abs. And all that these exercises require is your own body weight. No cables, pulleys, plates or gym memberships needed.

Free weights (barbell/dumbbell)

A set of dumbbells is a worthy investment. To start, one 10-lb pair for girls or 20 lbs for guys can fulfill your resistance requirements. With a set of dumbbells, you can perform shoulder presses, curls, triceps extensions, rows, squats and flies. A fitness ball allows you to incorporate chest exercises as well. It is also great for core strength training.

Cross training

In order to achieve full fitness, you should regularly engage in all three activities – strength, stamina and stretching. To let one area predominate is to allow your physicality to suffer and to court injury. The inveterate runner often lacks strength and falls prey to hip and knee ailments. The weightlifter finds his bulky muscles tight and inflexible, which gives rise to neck pain and headaches. If he doesn't cross train, the lungs and heart of the yogi may be as poorly conditioned as his muscles are limber.

Cross training is great way of including a variety of activities into your weekly schedule while minimizing risk of injury and maximizing versatility. Injury can be easy if your only aerobic outlet is running or jumping rope, but by adding non-impact activities (biking, swimming or climbing stairs) you spare your joints while working different muscles. The variations are limited only by your imagination. Find a set of stairs nearby, and climb as many flights as you can. Do a set of sit-ups or pushups before you descend. Or locate your nearest hill and jog or walk to the top. Leave a jump rope at the top of the hill and skip to the length of your favorite song. Then do a set of sit-ups or pushups before going back to the bottom. Go to your local track, run a lap, do a set of pushups and repeat. (Four laps equal a mile.) Better still, invent a routine of your own and mail it in to contact@adamdavemd.com.

Whether it's running, riding, surfing, playing pick-up basketball, gardening, whatever, the goal is simply to get out and have fun. Calorie burn is merely a nifty perk.

FITNESS TEST

Now that we've discussed physical activity, how do you assess how physically fit you are?

Why, with the physical fitness test, as the name suggests. The physical fitness test is popular among the armed forces, which use it as a minimum standard for physical testing and measurement. Variations exist, but generally the fitness test consists of a timed run and as many push-ups (or pull-ups) and sit-ups as you can do. This simple test does a fine job of quickly assessing upper body strength, core power and stamina.

In the army, the test consists of a timed 2-mile run, followed by timed push-ups and timed sit-ups. Each event is scored on a scale of 100. Here are the maximum and minimum scores:

2-mile run
> maximum: 13 minutes (men); 15:36 (women)
> minimum: 15:54 (men); 18:54 (women)

Push-ups (2 minute time-limit)
> maximum: 71 (men); 42 (women, on knees)
> minimum: 42 (men); 19 (women, on knees)

Sit-ups (2 minute time-limit)
> maximum: 78 (men and women)
> minimum: 53 (men and women)

The marines use pull-ups instead of push-ups, with 3 pull-ups, 50 crunches and 3 miles in 28:00 minutes set as the minimum. Maximum is 20, 100 and 18:00, respectively.

The navy seals use running, push-ups, pull-ups, sit-ups and swimming.

The President's Challenge Program, which includes an assessment of flexibility and of body composition, may be the most comprehensive of the variations and therefore best suited to our purposes. It includes a 1.5-mile run, half sit-ups, push-ups and a sit-and-reach test (to measure flexibility).

By performing a fitness test, you can assess your level and use it to chart your progress as your activity increases and your nutrition improves. If you'd like to see how your fitness compares to that of others, visit www.adultfitnesstest.org and record your scores to be assigned a percentile rank.

Knowing how fast you can run a mile or two should be as common as knowing your telephone number or address. It's part of your personal identification and makes you unique. Slow or fast, you're you and there's no one else like you.

My Fitness

Stamina (1.5 mile run):
Strength
        half sit-ups:
        pushups:
Sit-and-reach test:

COURSE FIVE: THE PARADIGM LIFE

Now that we have applied the scientific approach to the realms of fitness and nutrition, we can briefly examine the other areas of life and do the same with each.

Really, the scientific method is one of the finest methods mankind has devised for separating truth from illusion. In other words, it tells you what is there from what you think you see there. Is that an oasis we see, or is it really water? In order to really take a sip, we first must subject it to the test of our senses. By reasoning scientifically we are able to shed light on any observable phenomenon, be it as complex as the DNA double helix or as simple as your diet. Though you may have learned it in school and just as quickly forgotten it, you use the scientific method in daily life all the time, even though you may not realize it.

The method involves these steps:

1. Make an observation.

Example pertaining to diet: *My stomach hurts whenever I eat things like sandwiches, pizza or bagels.*

2. Invent a tentative description, called a hypothesis, which is consistent with what you have observed.

Example: *All these darn foods are made with bread. Maybe it is the bread that makes me bloated and backed up.*

3. Use the hypothesis to make predictions.

Example: *Bread is a grain. If I ate other types of grains, I'd feel bloated too.*

4. Test those predictions by experiments or further observations and modify the hypothesis in light of your results.

Example: *I also experience bloat when I eat pasta and noodles, but yesterday when I went for Chinese food, I ate brown rice, which is also a grain, and I felt okay. So not all grains upset my stomach.*

Alternative hypothesis: *Noodles and bread share the same ingredient: wheat. Maybe I am sensitive to wheat.*

5. Make and test additional predictions. Repeat steps 3 and 4 until there are no discrepancies between prediction and observation.

Example: *Looking on the ingredients list, I notice that many soy products contain wheat. If indeed I am sensitive to wheat and eat a soy burger, then I should feel bloated. This turns out to be the case. However, soy products also happen to be among the most common food allergens. Maybe I am sensitive to soy as well. I find that I cannot tolerate tofu very well, even if it is organic. But tempeh, which is fermented soy, causes me no problems. Hmmm...*

6. Derive a conclusion.

Example: *I am sensitive to wheat products and to some types of soy. I'd do best to avoid wheat altogether and to cut down on soy.*

This conclusion has withstood your experiments and now can be called a theory, which you can apply to your life and amaze your friends the next time you go out for Italian food, or Mexican, or Chinese, etc., as chances are some of your near and dear are among the millions that are wheat sensitive, though they may not know it yet.

In such a way, you can use a scientific approach to life to shed light on each of the three components of who you are: body, mind and soul.

BODY

The components of a healthy body are diet, exercise and rest/recovery.

1. *Diet*

As we have proved, plants are the healthiest foods around. Raw and lightly-cooked **sweets** (fruit), **greens** (vegetables), and **beans** (legumes) should make up your entire diet, with some **seeds** (flax, chia) for omega-3s.

2. *Exercise*

Reasoning scientifically, we have covered the components of physical fitness (body composition, activity, maximum activity) and determined ideal body weight, body fat percentage and activity level. We introduced you to the fitness test so that you may chart your progress. Remember, in the race of you against you, there are no losers. You always win.

3. *Rest and recovery*

Rest: Get a good night's sleep. Sleep improves memory, maintains a healthy weight, focuses concentration, regulates blood pressure and strengthens the immune system. And 7 to 9 hours of quality sleep per night meets the needs of most. If you engage in long bouts of strenuous exercise, you may require even more. If you're tired during the day, your quantity or quality of sleep is likely lacking. Reserve the bed for sleep and sexual intercourse only (that is, if your parents say coitus is okay). No eating, studying or watching TV permitted. It will just make you restless. Excessive body weight can cause sleep disorders, so please: Be lean.

Recovery: By recovery we refer to stretching and massage.

Stretch

Ever wonder why some old (and not so old) folks appear so stiff and bent-over? Years of moving through the limited range of motion that daily activities require trains our muscles to function only within that limited range. To counteract the abuse that results from poor posture, sitting at a desk, on a couch, or in the car, even lying in bed, it's important to work your muscles through a full range of motion, every day. In other words, stretch. Observe animals in nature, or your dog or cat. You'll notice that not a day goes by that they don't do some form of effortless elongation. There are even famous yoga postures named after them. *Downward dog*, anyone?

Massage

Massage is an excellent way to relieve trigger points.

What are those? you ask.

Commonly known as knots or kinks, trigger points are areas of contraction and irritability within muscles that have been over-worked or injured - as by falls, overexertion, or everyday activities like carrying a purse or operating a mouse. Trigger points can cause local pain or they may send pain and paresthesias (numbness, tingling) to distant sites of the body. This causes stiffness, muscle aches, joint pain and irritation of surrounding muscles.

Most cases of chronic pain, especially in the neck, shoulder, hip and knee, are due to trigger points. Unfortunately, most go undiagnosed or misdiagnosed as arthritis, herniated discs, tendinitis, etc. These serious conditions, once diagnosed or misdiagnosed often require treatment with medications and invasive surgical techniques. Much ado about *knothing*, or a knot-thing, we say.

Everybody has trigger points to some degree, even kids. Child athletes most commonly have them in the neck. Trigger points can be caused by a condition known as *Morton's Toe*, in which the second metatarsal (base of the toe) is longer than the first. Morton's Toe can cause poor posture, loss of balance and a tendency to fall.[100]

Through self-applied massage, you can easily eliminate trigger points, thereby regaining lost function, preventing injuries and assuring a lifetime of successful performance in the game of life. All you need is a good book,[101] your fingers and perhaps another massage tool such as a lacrosse ball, Thera Cane or foam roller.

MIND

The components of a healthy mind are reading, writing, thinking/problem solving and meditation/relaxation. Let's take each in turn.

4. *Reading*

Reading allows you to travel to distant lands from the comfort of your favorite armchair. It exercises your eyes, trains and focuses your mind, adds color to your imagination and improves verbal communication skills. Aim to read one journal (examples: *Time*, *National Geographic*, or *Runner's World*) per week and two books per month, one fiction and one nonfiction. You're almost done with this book and can cross it off your list.

5. *Writing*

Journal writing fosters introspection and creativity. It is time you spend with yourself. Whether it is to review the day's events, plan tomorrow's activities, write a letter to a loved one or jot down random thoughts, writing is a form of psychotherapy, where the author plays both therapist and patient. There is much to be gained from putting pen to paper, and much to be lost: Those who write down what they eat lose more weight and are more successful maintaining a healthy weight than those who don't. So buy a journal or start a blog and get to writing.

6. *Thinking/problem solving*

This may come on the job or in school. Or you may enjoy pursuits such as crossword puzzles, chess, Scrabble or other games. The mind likes to be trained. Use it or lose it.

7. *Meditation/relaxation*

Spend time in nature, take an early morning stroll, or sit in silence and watch your racing thoughts until they become still and disappear entirely. Focus on your breathing, take in some lovely scenery. Five to thirty minutes every day is all you need. If you fall asleep, it's a sign you're pretty relaxed – or that you need to catch up on some shut-eye! And remember, meditation can be performed while working out. On your next run, simply listen to your breathing and become entranced! Stillness in motion: What a rush!

SOUL

The components of a healthy spiritual life are loving relationships, service to others and artistic expression. Volumes of books have been written on each of these important topics, but for our purposes a few properly-chosen descriptive words suffice.

8. *Loving relationships*

Each day, spend some time with someone you care about. And tell that person how much she means to you. If you live alone, pick up the phone, pay a visit or invest in a pet.

9. *Service to others*

Service can come in the form of volunteering, for example at charitable events. Coach a Little League team, get involved in your local church or shelter. Remember, however, that charity begins at home. Make a meal for your loved ones or give some good advice to a friend in need. We are all connected. Helping others is helping yourself.

10. *Artistic expression*

Be it playing an instrument, writing a song or story, taking dance (or sculpting or painting) lessons, make an effort to express yourself artistically each week. Art in its purest form has no practical value (it won't drive you to the market or cure cancer): Its sole purpose is enjoyment, for both the creator and the observer.

AU REVOIR

Congratulations! You have made a meal of *The Paradigm Diet*. It is quite a mouthful, we recognize, but if you have *assimilated* even a small portion, you can be assured that know more about nutrition than most doctors and are surely able to prepare healthier meals than many 5-star chefs.

In our course on applied nutrition, we've learned how the human digestion works. We've studied the major nutrients, their functions and how they are handled by the body. We hope that you are convinced of what constitutes the healthiest diet on the planet, and confident of how to prepare meals in a way that is easy, affordable and enhances taste and nutrition.

We have also covered fitness and touched on your ideal body composition and activity level. You have taken an introspective look at the *diet* of your life and are welcome to submit your dietary assessment for a personalized evaluation.

The Paradigm Diet, a raw and lightly-cooked total-plant diet, is the ideal cuisine for *homo sapiens* (you and me). **Together we can heal the world, one delicious bite at a time.**

Remember this: Even if in your own life you are far from Paradigm, any step you take towards perfection, however small, is a step in the right direction. So start now.

Seriously. Start now!

Eat fruit and only fruit for breakfast. Eat it throughout the day. And eat lots of it!

Once you feel your vitality surge, see if you can extend fruit consumption through lunch and to dinner. Ravaged by cravings? Have fruit. Feel tired? Choose fruit. Thirsty? Munch on sweet, juicy fruit.

Then, revise your evening meal so that vegetables (particularly greens) and vegetable fruits (tomatoes, cucumbers, bell peppers, olives and avocados) make up at least half the plate, with the other half consisting of beans, potatoes or both.

Finally, increase your physical activity.

Then, let all else follow.

If you falter, you have not failed.

The more you let plants predominate, the more perfect is your diet, the more you heal the planet, and the more peaceful we are as a people.

Plants. Planet. People. Peace. Practice makes Paradigm. Live it! Love it! Make it your own!

DESSERT: DIETARY ASSESSMENT

The word *diet* commonly refers to the food you eat, especially as part of a weight-loss regimen, and may invoke painful memories and images of restriction and suffering. Let's pull ourselves outside of the box. As we shall see, the broader definition of the word includes everything you take in and experience repeatedly.

Diet derives from the Middle English *diete*, from Latin *diaeta*, from Greek *diaita*, and ultimately from *diaitasthai*, meaning **to lead one's life.**

Literally, your diet is your manner of living, or your lifestyle. It is who you are, and you are not only what you eat, but where you go, whom you spend time with, what you do and how you think and feel.

This dietary assessment is an exercise in introspection. It has intrinsic value, which means that the benefit resides in filling it out. It will clarify your lifestyle, identify your personal goal and assist you in achieving it, provided you are honest and thorough. In fact, the next hour promises to be one of the most important hours of your life – provided you are honest and thorough.

Please be completely honest and thorough.

As you complete the questionnaire, you'll notice that some of the questions have answers that are assigned numerical values. For these, choose the number that corresponds to your answer, and at the end of the assessment, tally your score. To see where you stand, or sit, or fit. You get the drift.

A. Personal Information
Name:
Age:
Email:
Today's date:
Birthday:
Birth time/place:

I. Goal
1. Which of the following is MOST important to you? (*choose only one*)
[ ] Weight loss
      - How many lbs?
      - By what date?
[ ] Increased energy
[ ] Better overall fitness and muscle tone
[ ] Get better grades
[ ] Do better in sports
[ ] Clear up my complexion
[ ] Pain relief (specify):
[ ] Make better food choices
[ ] Eliminate food cravings, sensitivities and allergies
[ ] Reverse chronic illness(es):
[ ] Decrease my medication (specify):
[ ] Overcome addiction (specify):
[ ] Raise healthier kids (*you may also choose another*)

II. Vital statistics
2. Current weight:
3. Adults - weight when you reached your adult height:
4. What do you think is your ideal weight?
5. Do you own a scale? Y (**1**) N (**0**)
6. When (date) was the last time you weighed yourself?
7. Circle how often you weigh yourself: once a year (**-1**), once per month (**0**), once weekly (**1**)
8. Please use a tape measure to record the following values:
Height (without shoes):
Hips (at widest point):
Wrist measurement (where your wrist bends):
Waist measurement (at narrowest point):
Neck:

BMI:[102]
My BMI is between 17 and 22 (**1**), between 23 and 25 (**0**), above 25 (**-1**)
BFP:[103]
My BFP is between 1 and 19 (**1**), between 20 and 29 (**0**), above 29 (**-1**)

III. Personal history
9. Relationship status: married/spoken for (**1**), single/dating (**0**), divorced/bereaved (**-1**)
10. Kids/ages:

11. Type of work/grade in school:

12. Hours per week:

13. Do you drive or take the bus to work/school?
If yes, daily commute in minutes (round trip):

14. Most of my day is spent sitting (**-1**)/standing(**0**)/walking(**1**)

IV. Medical history
15. Date you were last seen by a physician:

16. Reason for visit:

17. Menstrual cycle (if applicable)
      Average length:
      Regular/irregular
      Age at menarche (first period)
      Age at menopause (if applicable)

Medications (list all)

18. prescription: Y(**-1**) N (**1**)

19. non-prescription (include supplements):

20. multivitamin? Y(**1**), N(**0**)

21. Medical conditions (list all):
22. On a weekly basis, I suffer (mark all that apply):
[ ] Migraines/headaches
[ ] Asthma/breathing difficulty
[ ] Acne/eczema
[ ] Gas/bloat/stomach upset
[ ] Diarrhea/constipation
[ ] Fatigue
[ ] Bad breath
[ ] Body odor
[ ] Sleep difficulties
[ ] Excessive mucus
23. List any conditions that run in your immediate family:

V. Diet

24. Which term most closely describes you?
[ ] vegan (**3**)
[ ] vegetarian (**2**) (if so, do you eat milk or eggs?)
[ ] pescatarian (**1**)
[ ] omnivore (a little of everything) (**0**)
[ ] carnivore (meat at most meals) (**-1**)
[ ] junk food addict (**-2**)
[ ] other (please describe):
25. How many calories do you eat a day (you may "guesstimate")?

26. How many grams of protein do you eat each day?
a. less than 50 grams
b. more than 50 grams
c. don't know/care
27. How many times do you eat out (restaurants, cafeteria, deli/grocery, salad bar, take-out)?
a. more than once per day (**-2**)
b. once per day (**-1**)
c. more than once per week but not every day (**0**)
d. rarely, if at all (**1**)

Complete the following sentences
28. MOST of my meals are prepared by me/a loved one (**1**)/a personal chef/housekeeper (**0**)/a stranger (**-1**).

29. I eat most of my meals alone/with company.

30. On average, it takes me more than(**1**)/less than (**0**)20 minutes to consume a meal.

31. I chew each mouthful more than(**1**)/less than (**0**)20 times.

32. MOST of my meals are eaten:
Raw/Steamed/Boiled/Sautéed (**1**)
Broiled/Baked/Fried/Microwaved (**-1**)

33. At the market, which section do you spend the most time in? produce (**1**), packaged (**0**), meat (**-1**)

34. Which section do you spend the most money in? produce (**1**), packaged (**0**), meat (**-1**)

35. Where do you do most of your grocery shopping?

36. How much is your weekly grocery bill?

37. Do you like to cook? Y(**1**), N(**-1**)
If so, what is your favorite dish to make?

38. Name your favorite:
fruit:
vegetable:
legume:

dish:
snack:
cuisine:

39. How often do you use a microwave? Daily (**-1**) Weekly (**0**) Never (**1**)

40. Do you own a blender?

41. Do you smoke cigarettes? Y(**-1**) N(**1**) How many per day?

42. Do you use any illicit drugs (specify)? Y(**-1**) N(**1**)

43. Do you drink alcohol?
If yes, how many alcoholic drinks per week (one drink is 12 oz beer, 5 oz wine, or a 1.5 oz shot of hard liquor)? More than 14 (**-1**) Between 7 and 14 (**0**) Less than 7 (**1**)

44. Do you drink coffee?
If yes, how many 5 oz cups per day? More than 2 (**-1**), 1 or 2 (**0**), None (**1**)
Sweetened? y/n (specify type)
Milk/milk substitute? y/n (specify type)

45. How many glasses of water do you drink a day (1 glass is 8 oz)? less than 4 (**-1**), 4 or more (**1**)
46. List other beverages you regularly consume:

47. What do you eat on a typical day? (if no day is typical, use yesterday; if you can't remember yesterday, go to www.fitday.com and record tomorrow's intake) **be specific, including portion size whenever possible**)
Breakfast:

Snack:

Lunch:

Snack:

Dinner:

Dessert:

48. How many servings of the following foods do you consume **per day**? Less than 10 (**-1**) Between 10 and 20 (**0**) 21 or more (**1**)
Vegetables (1 cup)
Fruit (1 cup, or 1 medium)
Beans (1/2 cup)
49. How many servings **per day**? More than 4 (**-1**) Less than 4 (**0**) None (**1**)
Nuts (serving size is 1 oz, or 20 nuts)
Grains (bread, rice, pasta, cereal, etc.)
Fast food/fried food
Salty snacks
Sweets/desserts (including dark chocolate)
Soft drinks
50. How many servings (**per week**)? More than 10 (**-1**) Less than 10 (**0**) None (**1**)

Meat
Dairy
Eggs
Fish

Peanuts/tree nuts
Corn
Soy
Wheat

51. Name the three packaged foods you eat most (packaged is anything in a box, bag, bottle or can, not including fruits, vegetables, beans, water or condiments).
1.
2.
3.

52. List your three favorite spices.

53. Do you cook with/use oil? Y (-1) N (1)
54. How often do you read labels? most of time(1)/some of time(0)/not at all(-1)

55. How often do you buy organic produce? Most of time(1)/some of time(0)/not at all(-1)
56. Have you ever sprouted or grown your own food? Y(1)N(0)(specify)

Take this short quiz:
57. Which food has the most protein, per calorie.
[ ] Whole wheat bread
[ ] Filet mignon
[ ] Lentils
[ ] Spinach

58. Which food has the most cholesterol?
[ ] Olive oil
[ ] Soybeans
[ ] One large chicken breast
[ ] One large egg

59. List the food with the most fiber (per calorie).
[ ] Raspberries
[ ] Oatmeal
[ ] Spinach
[ ] Chicken breast
[ ] Walnuts

60. Circle one source of vitamin D.
cheese/spinach/sunlight/avocado
61. Circle one source of vitamin B12.
nutritional yeast/garbanzo beans/whole grain bread

62. Which food has the most calcium (per calorie)?
a. Milk
b. Spinach
c. Beef
d. Garbanzo beans

Answers: 57. Spinach 58. Egg 59. Raspberries 60. Sunlight 61. Nutritional yeast 62. Spinach
For each correct answer give yourself 1 point.

63. How many grams of fiber do you eat per day?
Less than 25 grams (**-1**)
Between 25 and 50 grams (**0**)
More than 50 grams (**1**)

VI. Lifestyle
64. How many days per week do you exercise? None (**-1**) Less than 4 (**0**) 4 or more (**1**)
65. How many minutes per week? Less than 3 hours (**-1**) More than 3 hours (**1**)

66. List the exercises you do on a weekly basis?
67. Which do you prefer, the gym or outdoors?

68. Rank each exercise in order of preference:
[ ] strength (weights, resistance)
[ ] stamina (cardio)
[ ] stretching (yoga, Pilates, massage)

69. If you could only do one exercise, which would it be?

70. Hours of sleep per night: less than 7 (**-1**) more than 7 (**1**)
71. Do you keep a journal? Y(**1**)N(**-1**)   If so how often?

72. How many times **per week** do you brush your teeth? Less than 7 (**-1**) 7 or more (**1**)   Floss? Less than 7 (**-1**) 7 or more (**1**)
73. How many hours of TV do you watch **per week**? Less than 7 (**1**) 7 to 10 (**0**) More than 10 (**-1**)
74. When and where was your last vacation?

75. When was the last book you read *cover to cover*? Over a month ago (**-1**) Within the past month (**1**)
76. When was the last time you went either to the beach or to a park? Over a week ago (**-1**) Within the past week (**1**)
77. How many minutes do you spend each week in direct sunlight? Under 1 hour (**-1**) More than 1 hour (**1**)
78. How many bowel movements do you have **per week**? Less than 7 (**-1**) Between 7 and 10 (**0**) At least 10 (**1**)
79. Do you have Morton's toe? y/n/don't know

VII. Rewrite the goal you listed at the beginning of this questionnaire.

80. On a scale of 1-10, 1 being not at all, 10 being **the most important thing in the world**, how important is it to you to achieve this goal?
1   2   3   4   5   6   7   8   9   10

If you did not choose 7 or higher, name a goal that is more important to you:

81. On a scale of 1-10, how confident are you in your ability to achieve this goal?
1   2   3   4   5   6   7   8   9   10

If your confidence is not a 7 or higher, take a moment and modify your goal to make its accomplishment more attainable.
Rewrite you goal here:

SCORE CARD

If you scored:
-21 to -40: *Help, we're dying!* your insides are screaming. Seriously, your habits are in the red. Shape up or a hospital admission awaits – if you're lucky. The coroner is not far.

-1 to -20: Er, there is room for improvement. As in, several hundred pages of room. As in, reread this book. The second time around will often result in a substantially better score.

0 to 24: not bad; but not great either. In other words, average. You're on the right track, but we know you can do better!

25 to 50: your *diet* - and all that makes it up - is pretty snazzy. You've read and applied the Paradigm Principles. Congrats and keep it up!

APPENDIX A: PARADIGM STEPS

All it takes to go from *processed* to *Paradigm* are these 3 easy steps.

1. Assess

Start by determining your current caloric intake. Go to fit-day.com or nutridiary.com and sign up for a free membership (or enter as a guest). The USDA has a database of foods that you can use, available at www.nal.usda.gov.

What you need to do is track, for a period of 24 hours, exactly what goes in your mouth. Sun up to sun up. Do this on a weekend, so work and other obligations won't get in the way. Every food and fluid that you ingest you must record.

Don't change your diet because it is being recorded. This is called the Hawthorne effect, in which subjects in an experiment act differently than they do in real life simply because they know they're being watched. It messes up the results, and because this is your experiment, accuracy is important.

The goal is to get a realistic understanding of where your diet is. You'll get a lot of information from this simple exercise, including how much of the recommended intake of each nutrient you consume. What we are concerned with are three things: total calories, total fiber and total water. Really, only one thing matter, and that's fiber. Because as your fiber intake goes up, your water intake follows, and your total caloric intake is lower than it otherwise would be.

What to expect

At first you will be bothered that you have an assignment that involves recording and computing.

Then you will be annoyed that you have to measure servings and look up ingredients. You may be tempted to avoid eating altogether just to save yourself the hassle. Resist this temptation. Eat as you normally do. Remember, this is only one day.

Finally, you will be intrigued and enlightened as you find out what you were eating and exactly what is in your food. You'll be impressed by the pie graphs and other cool applications available on these free, user-friendly sites.

Where to go from here

As we said, calories matter less than water and fiber intake, which go hand in hand. You should be getting at least 8 glasses per day of water in food. That's 2 liters. At least. Thirty grams of fiber is the absolute minimum. If you are not achieving 2 L of water and 30 g of fiber in your food, you're not alone. Remember, the average person consumes a paltry 10 grams of fiber and only 20 percent of water from food. So don't worry, you'll get better. That's what steps 2 and 3 are for.

2. Introduce

Start the next day with 1 or 2 glasses of water. This will clean your stomach of any residue from the previous night's meal, as well as dilute stomach acid. It may even bring about a bowel movement. (Gastrocolic reflex, remember?)

Then, eat only fruit for breakfast. If you are not in the habit of eating breakfast, try blending a shake. Simply fill up your blender with these 3 ingredients: 1 cup juicy fruit, 1 cup frozen berries, 1 banana. Then drink it down and say, *Ahhhhh!* (The *Ahhhhh!* is, of course, optional.)

If your normal breakfast consists of things such as eggs, toast, cereal, pizza or ice cream, etc., replace them with fruit. Start with juicy fruits (melons, citrus) and move to more concentrated fruit (bananas, dates) later in the morning if your hunger is not satisfied. See yourself as a kid in the candy store, surrounded by colorful sweets that you can eat to your heart's content.

Eat only fruit until noon, as much or as little as you wish. Carry some with you to work or to school. Keep some in your bag, at your desk, and/or in the car.

Don't feel guilty if you have 6 bananas. There is no limit to how much fruit you can enjoy. Actually, there is a limit, but your body will tell you before you reach it.

What to expect

If for breakfast you usually eat fatty, salty foods, you may initially be bothered by cravings. This is because old habits die hard. We are hard-wired to crave fat and eat a lot of it. It's an evolutionary consequence of living through famines. Famines are history. Now it's time to feast. On fruit. Remember, the real craving is for sweet food, the taste bud for which is on the tip of the tongue, as if to say: Gimme more!

If you usually skip breakfast and fill yourself up on coffee, you may find that you are not hungry in the morning. Start by reducing coffee intake to 2 cups at most, and eating 1 piece of sweet fruit. Just one. Or as mentioned, make a shake. Then see how you feel. In all likelihood, sweet succulent fruit will awaken your appetite. Then as you begin eating more fruit and transitioning to bananas and dates without guilt, you will find you quite enjoy this change. You have more energy, can eat a lot more, and fill up the toilet more than ever before.

You will likely notice weight loss. That is, if you need to lose weight. However, some experience initial weight gain, especially if you undertake an exercise regimen. This is because exercise increases blood volume (water in your veins) and bone density. Even if you add pounds, your body fat content is going down. To verify, measure your waist and watch it shrink.

Stay on the fruit till noon kick for a month or so, at least.

You may even wish to eat only fruit and perhaps some raw vegetables through lunch.

Stay here for another month or so, at least, before moving on to Step 3.

3. Substitute

After you've come to enjoy eating fruit for breakfast and maybe even for lunch, it is time to make healthy substitutions. The trick is to phase in greens, beans and maybe some seeds and phase out other foods. Let's list them: meat, dairy and eggs. You see, the list isn't really that long. Reduce consumption of grains and nuts in favor of sweets, greens, beans and seeds.

What to expect

This is when the food cravings attack head on. But they won't be all that bad now that you've reset your taste buds by eating unseasoned fruit. And remember, by choosing vegetables, you can eat much larger quantities than you ever could by making a meal of meat and bread. And your body loves bulk. Take consolation in this fact. You may now eat as much as you wish, guilt-free.

Start your evening meal with several pieces of vegetables (bell pepper, cucumbers, mushroom, tomatoes, carrots, snap peas, celery) or perhaps a large salad. In other words, dice these vegetables and scatter them over a bowl of lettuce, dress with lemon, salt, yeast and maybe some Tabasco.

Then take your steamer and add any combination of the following: potatoes, broccoli, kale, green beans, Brussels sprouts. Steam for the recommended time, which is almost always 5 minutes, except in the case of potatoes, which require 5 minutes more. Add olives, garlic, avocado and beans, as much or as little as you wish. You will never get tired of this evening meal. But if you do, remember your healthy substitutions:

If you crave meat, have beans.

If you crave nuts, have seeds.

If you crave cheese, have tofu or nutritional yeast.

If you crave bread, have potatoes, sweet potatoes, squash or bananas.

Say it aloud. "Meat beans. Nuts seeds. Cheese yeast. Bread bananas." Say it until the associations stick.

Use nutritional yeast, tofu and coconut milk more liberally at first, as they impart a savory taste that at first you might miss when removing animal protein and processed grains from your diet.

Be patient with yourself. It may take months to completely phase out the empty foods. Remember, Rome wasn't built in a day. You are an architect for lasting change, and your body is the edifice, so make it a palace.

Remember that your transition to a plant-based diet is the single greatest contribution you will ever make to the health not only of your body but also of the environment and economy. In fact, the whole world depends on you!

That's it. We're done. You're done. The New You is here. Welcome, friend.

APPENDIX B: ELEVEN MYTHS

You shouldn't eat late at night. Your body will just store the food as fat.

In fact, the opposite is true. It's *best* to make your evening meal the biggest of the day. When you consume food, you activate your parasympathetic nervous system. This is the housekeeping arm of your autonomic nervous system that conserves energy and metabolizes food. In other words, it helps you *rest and digest.*

By contrast, input from the sympathetic nervous system is responsible for your *fight or flight* response. It is active during the day as you face challenges, meet deadlines and argue with the phone company.

These two arms, sympathetic and parasympathetic, oppose each other. In other words, the stresses of the day interfere with digestion and with the functions of the parasympathetic, which is most effective when your body is at rest.

Small portions are best. Don't ever stuff yourself.

This is only true if you eat high-fat animal products and refined carbohydrates, which are so loaded with calories that if you don't restrict yourself to palm-sized portions you can easily overeat. Sweets, greens, beans and seeds, on the other hand, are nutritionally dense rather than calorically dense, and they are so high in water and fiber that you can eat your fill while taking in a fraction of the calories present in even one slice of pizza. In reality, small meals throughout the day can deplete your body's digestive enzymes and delay the passage of food through your intestines. This can lead to stomach upset, gas and bloat. Your stomach functions most efficiently when it is full. As it has a capacity of over 3 L, equivalent to 12 8-oz glasses of water, full means a lot of food. In fact, more food than you are likely accustomed to consuming, so rather than *restrain* yourself from eating too much, you'll have to *train* yourself to eat enough! It's okay to go to bed with a full belly. If your meal is nutritious, when you wake up in the morning your stomach will be flat as a board.

It's wise to drink a lot of water.

Sure, water is good to drink, but your main source of H_2O should not be by the glass. Drinking large amounts of liquids, especially with meals, can dilute enzymes and increase the work of digestion. Also, many brands of drinking water - not just tap water but also bottled versions - are known to contain high levels of metals, chemicals and other pollutants, including bacteria. It is best to satisfy your hydration requirements through food. By weight, fruits and vegetables are 80 percent or more water. A diet that emphasizes these foods can easily meet 80 percent or more of your recommended water intake. And the water in plant foods is in its purest possible form, naturally filtered through their roots, stems and leaves. So, eat up!

Milk does a body good.

It is true that milk is high in calcium and vitamin D and that these nutrients are needed for strong bones. But drinking milk can actually weaken your bones. How can this be? Milk is high in animal protein and acid-forming. To buffer the excess acid produced by protein digestion, your body borrows calcium from its storage site in your bones, leading to osteoporosis and increasing your risk for broken bones as you age. Leafy green vegetables are higher in calcium than milk, and your best source of vitamin D is your own skin, which produces it on exposure to the sun.

Besides, no animal other than humans consumes the milk of another species, let alone drinks milk into adulthood. Two-thirds of the population is unable to digest milk, which can result in abdominal cramps, bloat, gas and other more serious conditions. Mother's milk is for babies. Cow's milk is for baby cows.

Animal foods (meat, eggs, dairy) are highest in protein.

Indeed, animal foods are high in protein, but they contain little else of nutritional value. They lack water, are devoid of fiber and vitamin C and contain large amounts of cholesterol, fat and saturated fat. The vitamins and minerals animal foods do contain come by way of the plants they consume. Plants, not animals, are the ultimate source of nutrients, including vitamins, minerals and even protein.

The protein in animal products contributes to cancer, weight gain, osteoporosis and kidney stones. Per calorie, leafy green vegetables contain more protein than meat, and beans are also high in protein. A diet that includes generous helpings of these lovely foods easily provides adequate protein to meet the needs of even the most active and actively growing persons.

Olive oil is good for you.

Oils are highly processed foods. Like white sugar, they have no vitamins, minerals, water or fiber. Unlike sugar, oils are pure fat, and fat serves a very limited function in the diet. In fact, the digestion of fat produces free radicals, which contribute to cancer and premature aging. In other words, the more fat in your diet, the more free-radical damage, and the older you look.

Whole foods – fruits, vegetables, beans and seeds – contain adequate amounts of fat, including the essential fatty acids. Even those foods commonly considered fat-free, such as lemons and onions, contain fat. Added fat in the form of oil, butter, margarine or lard, not to mention animal products such as chicken and beef, is unnecessary and can even be deadly.

To fulfill your fat cravings, choose olives, avocados, tofu and even a little coconut milk over oils and nuts.

Nuts are healthy fats.

Nuts are high in the pro-inflammatory omega-6 fatty acids, which contribute to conditions including asthma, arthritis, heart disease and chronic pain. Nuts are also concentrated foods devoid of water, which makes them very hard to digest. Avoid nuts and instead choose seeds such as flax and chia seeds, which are high in anti-inflammatory omega-3 fatty acids. These fats oppose the actions of omega-6, protect the heart and offer pain relief.

A healthy diet should include several servings per day of whole grains.

So says the USDA. Sadly, the Department of Agriculture has vested interests. In fact, 20 percent of government food subsidies is devoted to the production of grains (in contrast to only 2 percent for legumes, and less than 1 percent for fruits and vegetables).

In reality, grain products are not health foods. Whether refined or whole, grains such as wheat, barley, rye and possibly oats are a major cause of food allergies and sensitivities. Like nuts, grains are high in pro-inflammatory omega-6 fats and acid-forming. Also, whole grains have high glycemic values and are low in fiber relative to vegetables and beans. This makes eating grains a recipe for weight gain, which is why they are replacing grass as cow feed: To fatten up them and those who eat them.

Fruit is high in sugar.

Fruit derives most of its calories from simple sugars, which are rapidly assimilated to provide instant fuel your body depends on. In fact, your brain uses glucose almost exclusively. The water and fiber in fruits modulate the absorption of sugar into your bloodstream. This assures steady levels of energy. Though sweeter than candy, fruits are mostly low glycemic foods, meaning the sugar they contain does not play havoc with your blood sugar. Per serving, whole grains are much higher in carbohydrates than fruits. The carbohydrate in grains such as rice and pasta gets broken down to the same simple sugars – glucose and fructose – that make up fruit, making grains actually much higher in sugar. Want to reduce your sugar consumption and still satisfy your sweet tooth? Give up grains, which are not even sweet, and choose fruit.

I don't poop every day, but my doctor says I'm not constipated.

Untrue. Our digestive systems are all designed the same, consisting of 30 feet of tube from mouth to anus. Thirty feet. Ten times the length of your torso. The differences in our bowel habits arise from food choices. One word: fiber, or roughage, or bulk. Due to a diet generally higher in this *call it what you will*, vegetarians move food through the intestinal tract much more rapidly than meat-eaters, whose food can fester in the bowels for up to a week, fodder for unfriendly bacteria and foul-smelling to boot.

Going every day should be the rule. In fact, going several times per day is normal. Just observe infants, whose digestion is in perfect working order. They go after every feeding. If you have three meals a day, you should have at least as many daily BMs, no matter what your doctor says. Think large, soft bananas.

Remember, the human gastrointestinal tract is dependent on fiber, with intakes of greater than 30 grams per day necessary for optimal function. Because animal products contain no fiber, your intake of this important nutrient is inversely proportional to the amount of animal food you consume. **So beat the meat (and eggs and dairy) and eat more sweets (and greens and beans).**

Vegans require supplementation with vitamin B12, as they are likely deficient.

Actually, a large portion of the population is B12 deficient, as many as 30 percent of adults over age 60.[104] Only 1 percent of the American population is vegan, and so if 30 percent of the population has B12 deficiency, the majority - you guessed it - the majority consume animal products. In fact, *the likelihood a person is B12 deficient may actually increase with higher intakes of B12.*

How can this be?

Your dietary B12 requirement is very minimal. In fact, the amount of B12 you need in food is measured by the microgram, or thousandth of a milligram, which is one millionth of a gram. Which is very very small! This is because most of the B12 in your body gets recycled and used over and over again.[105] Also, bacteria in your colon produce it and other vitamins, which your body is able to absorb. So B12 deficiency is less likely to arise from inadequate intake than from defects in absorption. These defects can occur in the stomach, which produces a chemical (intrinsic factor) needed to absorb vitamin B12, or in the small intestine, the site of B12's entrance into your blood. Damage to the small intestine can result from an intolerance to wheat products; damage to the stomach may occur as a result of excessive amounts of acid produced by years of consuming animal products, whose digestion requires large amounts of acid. *In other words, eating foods high in B12 (animal foods) may result in B12 deficiency.*

So just being a vegan does not mean you need to supplement with vitamin B12, and if the statistics are any indication, avoiding animal products may offer you some protection from deficiency. A study in Japan found that vegan children on a diet of brown rice and Nori seaweed (an unreliable source of B12) all had B12 levels in the normal range.[106]

In truth, it is meat eating that poses the biggest risk of B12 deficiency. If you consume or have consumed animal products regularly, you may have already suffered damage to your stomach that results in inadequate absorption and should talk to your doctor about checking your B12 levels. Deficiency can produce symptoms of anemia (fatigue, anxiety, pale skin and rapid heart rate), in addition to numbness and tingling of the arms and feet and other nervous system abnormalities.

APPENDIX C: NUTRIENTS

As you can tell by now, our aim is to avoid focusing on particular nutrients in isolation. Whole foods provide a wide array of vitamins and minerals and the emphasis should therefore be on what you eat rather than what is in what you eat. However, we recognize that no book on nutrition would be complete without a list of nutrients, along with their functions and sources. So here goes.

But remember that in addition to these 30 or so essential nutrients, there are hundreds if not thousands of phytonutrients recently discovered and still undiscovered, which by definition exist only in plants. So eat your sweets. And your greens. And your beans. And your seeds.

And be well.

biotin: needed for healthy skin and energy production; sources include Swiss chard, tomatoes, carrots, cauliflower, onions, avocados, raspberries and bananas

calcium: strong bones, nerves and muscles; spinach, collards, basil, cinnamon, Swiss chard, kale, lettuce, celery, broccoli, cabbage, green beans, zucchini, garlic, tofu, Brussels sprouts, oranges, asparagus, crimini mushrooms

carotenoids: antioxidants; sweet potatoes, spinach, kale, collard greens, carrots, Swiss chard, winter squash, lettuce, cantaloupe, bell peppers, broccoli, asparagus, papaya, tomatoes, cayenne, green peas,

Brussels sprouts, grapefruit, green beans, watermelon, apricots, parsley, celery, olives, zucchini, figs

choline: nerve and muscle function; navy beans, Brussels sprouts, broccoli, pinto beans, kidney beans, cauliflower, asparagus, spinach, green peas, tofu, cabbage, crimini mushrooms, squash, avocado

chromium: normalizes blood sugar, cholesterol; Romaine lettuce, onions, tomatoes

coenzyme Q: antioxidant reactions, energy production; broccoli, cauliflower, oranges, strawberries

copper: anti-oxidant; crimini mushrooms, Swiss chard, spinach, kale, summer squash, asparagus, eggplant, tomatoes, green beans, potatoes, sweet potatoes, kiwi, tofu, bell peppers, winter squash, soybeans, lentils

fiber: bowel regularity, normal blood sugar and cholesterol; raspberries, cauliflower, collard greens, broccoli, Swiss chard, spinach, celery, cabbage, grapefruit, green beans, eggplant, cranberries, strawberries, bell peppers, dried peas, winter squash, kale, carrots, summer squash, lentils, Brussels sprouts, asparagus, black beans, green peas, pinto beans

folate: red blood cell production; Romaine lettuce, spinach, asparagus, collards, broccoli, cauliflower, beets, lentils, celery, Brussels sprouts, pinto beans, black beans, chickpeas, kidney beans, summer squash, navy beans, papaya, green beans, cabbage, bell peppers, green peas, lima beans, winter squash, tomatoes

iodine: required for the synthesis of thyroid hormones, which regulate growth, development, metabolism and reproductive function; iodized salt, canned beans, seaweed, sauces and seasonings

iron: oxygen transport, energy production; spinach, turmeric, Swiss chard, basil, cinnamon, Romaine lettuce, tofu, Shiitake mushrooms, green beans, parsley, kale, broccoli, Brussels sprouts, asparagus, soybeans, olives, lentils, celery, cabbage, kidney beans

magnesium: muscle relaxation, bone strength; Swiss chard, spinach, summer squash, broccoli, basil, cucumbers, flax seeds, green beans, celery, collard greens, kale, black beans, beets, tomatoes, pinto beans, tofu, crimini mushrooms

manganese: healthy bones, nerves, thyroid; cinnamon, Romaine lettuce, pineapple, spinach, turmeric, collard greens, raspberries, Swiss chard, kale, garlic, grapes, summer squash, strawberries, green beans, chickpeas, tofu, broccoli, beets, flax seeds, crimini mushrooms, cauliflower

molybdenum: increases antioxidant capacity of blood, helps metabolize drugs and toxins; legumes are the richest source of molybdenum

niacin: fat metabolism; crimini mushrooms, asparagus, tomatoes, summer squash, green peas, collard greens, carrots, broccoli, spinach, eggplant, cauliflower, winter squash, raspberries, kale

omega-3 fatty acid (ALA): anti-inflammatory, cell membrane fluidity; flax seeds, chia seeds, cauliflower, cabbage, Romaine lettuce, broccoli, Brussels sprouts, winter squash, tofu, summer squash, collard greens, spinach, kale, soybeans, strawberries, green beans

pantothenic acid (vitamin B5): fat and carbohydrate metabolism; crimini mushrooms, cauliflower, broccoli, tomatoes, strawberries, winter squash, collard greens, Swiss chard

phosphorus: healthy bones, energy production; soybeans, lentils, great northern beans, chickpeas, navy beans, pinto beans, kidney beans, lima beans, green peas, tofu, dates,

potassium: healthy muscles and nerves, normal blood pressure; Swiss chard, crimini mushrooms, spinach, Romaine lettuce, celery, broccoli, winter squash, tomatoes, collard greens, summer squash, eggplant, cantaloupe, green beans, Brussels sprouts, kale, carrots, beets, papaya, asparagus, basil, cucumbers, turmeric, bell peppers, cauliflower, apricots

selenium: antioxidant; crimini mushrooms, Shiitake mushrooms, tofu, garlic, broccoli, asparagus, spinach

sodium (chloride): fluid balance, blood volume, blood pressure, nerve conduction, nutrient absorption; salt, canned beans, seaweed, sauces and seasonings

vitamin A: healthy eyesight, immune function; carrots, spinach, kale, parsley, bell peppers, Romaine lettuce, Swiss chard, sweet potatoes, cayenne, collards, cantaloupe, winter squash, apricots, broccoli, tomatoes, asparagus, basil, green beans, Brussels sprouts, summer squash, grapefruit, watermelon, cucumbers, prunes

vitamin B1 (thiamin): nervous, muscle, heart function and energy metabolism; Romaine lettuce, asparagus, crimini mushrooms, spinach, green peas, tomatoes, eggplant, Brussels sprouts, celery, cabbage, watermelon, bell peppers, carrots, squash, green beans, broccoli, kale, black beans, pineapple, oranges

vitamin B2 (riboflavin): energy production; crimini mushrooms, spinach, Romaine lettuce, asparagus, Swiss chard, broccoli, collards, green beans, celery, kale, cabbage, strawberries, tomatoes, cauliflower, raspberries, Brussels sprouts, summer squash, green peas, plums

vitamin B6: nervous tissue, sugar metabolism; spinach, bell peppers, garlic, cauliflower, bananas, broccoli, celery, asparagus, cabbage, crimini mushrooms, kale, collards, Brussels sprouts, watermelon, Swiss chard, cayenne, turmeric, tomatoes, carrots, summer squash, cantaloupe, eggplant, Romaine lettuce

vitamin B12: blood cell production, nervous system health; unwashed vegetables, nutritional yeast, colonic bacteria

vitamin C: antioxidant, iron absorption, anti-aging; bell peppers, parsley, broccoli, strawberries, cauliflower, lemon, Romaine lettuce, Brussels sprouts, papaya, kale, kiwi, cantaloupe, oranges, grapefruit, cabbage, tomatoes, Swiss chard, collards, raspberries, asparagus, celery, spinach, pineapples, green beans, summer squash

vitamin D: healthy bones and teeth, immune function, overall health; your skin is the best source, so get some sun!

vitamin E: antioxidant; Swiss chard, spinach, collard greens, kale, papaya, olives, bell peppers, Brussels sprouts, kiwi, blueberries, tomatoes, broccoli

vitamin K: blood clotting; bacteria in your colon produce vitamin K in adequate amounts to meet your metabolic needs; leafy greens are another source

zinc: immune function, metabolism; crimini mushrooms, spinach, summer squash, asparagus, chard, collards, green peas, broccoli

APPENDIX D:
TEN REASONS TO EAT SWEETS

Consider for a moment all the countries of this vast and beautiful planet and you'll notice that every culture is defined by its cuisine.

The Italians have their pasta, the French their pate, the Mexicans their tacos and tostadas.

The Chinese are known for their largely dairy-free, vegetable-centric diet, as well as for their low rates of many Western diseases, such as cancer, heart disease and strokes.

In fact, the Chinese eat **30 percent more calories** than the average American, and **weigh 20 percent less!**[107]

Speaking of America, as far as cuisine goes, what defines the most advanced nation in the world?

Two words: Fast food.

Or, if you prefer, one word:

McDonald's.

Or Wendy's.

Or KFC.

Etc.

Lacking its distinctive culinary dishes, America is fast adopting fast food as its fare of choice. The result is that more than two-thirds of the population is overweight. In fact, it is said that Europeans can spot American tourists not so much by their binoculars and colorful shirts but by the 30 or so extra lbs that the average Joe or Jane America carries around his waist (or her hips).

It is a shame that a nation priding itself on being the best in everything has a diet, with its reliance on processed grains and high-fat animal protein, that is by far the worst in the world!

It is high time that America adopts a diet to suit the ideals on which it was founded:

Life, not death.

Liberty, not slavery to empty-calorie foods.

The pursuit of happiness, not animal cruelty.

And while we're upgrading the American diet, why not shoot for the stars, and make the cuisine that defines this country the best out there?

The scientifically-proven healthiest diet is a whole food, plant-based diet that is high in water, fiber and other nutrients, and naturally low in calories, cholesterol and chemicals.

A diet rich in **sweets** (fruit), **greens** (veggies), **beans** and **seeds** is cost-effective and time-efficient. Not to mention that it spares the planet the pollution, pesticides and petroleum poured into the animals we savagely consume.

And so, here are ten reasons to adopt a whole-foods, plant-based diet. Or, if you prefer, the top reasons to eat less meat (and eggs and dairy) and more sweets (and beans and seeds).

I. If you eat meat, what you eat, EATS you.

1. Meat fills you up, and leaves you empty.

Though loaded with saturated fat, cholesterol and toxic chemicals, meat is low in most vitamins and minerals and contains little water and no fiber. The one nutrient it does have - animal protein - is linked to cancer, heart, bone and kidney disease. Humans can easily fulfill their daily protein requirement by eating only fruits and vegetables.

Take leafy greens, for instance. Calorie for calorie, spinach has more iron, calcium, protein and all major minerals than top sirloin. And spinach is filled with water, fiber and omega-3 fatty acids, without cholesterol or saturated fat.

2. Meat kills.

Animal protein is the root cause of cancer, heart disease and stroke, the top three killers in America, which makes meat, eggs and dairy the top three killers in America. 'Nuff said.

3. Meat is not meant for us.

Our earliest ancestors were predominately fruit eaters, as are our primate relatives (apes, gorillas), whose digestive systems most closely resemble our own. Animal protein makes up little if any of the caloric intake of these human-like species.

4. Dairy is to die for.

Cow's milk is indigestible by most humans and causes cancer (breast, prostate) and osteoporosis. It is also linked with autoimmune dysfunction, arthritis, acne, asthma, allergies, ear infections and kidney stones, among many other ailments. No animal drinks the milk of another species, or drinks it into adulthood, except humans. No animals suffer these same diseases, but us. Coincidence? Likely, not.

5. Eggs rot your heart.

Your body manufactures all the cholesterol it needs. Any dietary intake is by definition too much. In fact, excess cholesterol is deposited in the lining of the arteries supplying your heart and can give rise to heart attacks. The cholesterol in one egg (300 mg) can increase blood cholesterol by as much as 15 mg, and increase your risk for heart disease by 30 percent.[108] All animal foods contain cholesterol. Plant foods are naturally cholesterol-free. And let's face it, eggs stink both going in and coming out.

II. If you eat meat, what you eat, EATS the planet.

6. A meat feast causes worldwide famine.

The United Nations has recently recommended a global shift to a vegan diet. Meat eating is directly responsible for the water shortage, third world starvation and the greenhouse effect, in addition to deforestation and industrial pollution.[109]

To illustrate:

Eating one hamburger for lunch has 25 times the greenhouse effect as driving a car for a day. Over 5,000 gallons of water are required to produce 1 lb of beef. This is over 200 times the 25 gallons that go into a lb of lettuce.

Nearly fifteen times more land is used for growing hay for livestock than for growing vegetables. In countries where starvation is a reality, most of the agricultural land is used to raise livestock that the poor cannot afford. As a result, the number of **underfed and**

undernourished people in the world is now over 1 billion, which equals the number of those who by consuming excessive animal protein are **overfed and undernourished**.

Geophysicists estimate that if every American reduced meat consumption by just 20 percent, the greenhouse gas savings would be the same as if we all switched from a normal sedan to a hybrid Prius. That's a reduction in animal consumption of just one day per week.[110]

7. A meat-eater's pleasure comes by way of pain.

Animals raised for slaughter are robbed of their natural habitat and subjected to a savage cruelty that makes Hitler's concentration camps look like Club Meds.

Just because cows and pigs speak a language we cannot understand should not make us deaf to their cries of pain. In fact, the nerves of many animals are many times more sensitive than humans, which means they feel pain that is worse than our worst nightmares!

By eating chicken, beef, pork and fish, and even dairy and eggs (which are produced by subjecting animals to inhumane conditions) we participate in the misery of these unfortunate creatures and take in the toxic residues of the antibiotics, pesticides, hormones and fertilizers that make up their lives and their pain. Not only that, the stress hormone cortisol as well as other stress chemicals - including catecholamines such as adrenaline and norepinephrine - get released when an animal is slaughtered.[111] These powerful substances flood the bloodstream and surge into the animals' tissues. In humans, high levels of cortisol and catecholamines are associated with posttraumatic stress disorder and major depressive disorder,[112] conditions characterized by anxiety, difficulty concentrating, sadness, guilt and sleep difficulties. Side effects of excess cortisol include weight gain, a moon face and a buffalo hump. Not pretty.

It is not a great leap to argue that artificially elevating cortisol and catecholamine levels - by consuming foods rich in these chemicals - may exaggerate our own stress response, exacerbate these and other mood and anxiety conditions and even play a part in their etiology, or cause.

8. Meat eating bankrupts the economy.

US Healthcare is a 2.4 trillion dollar industry, of which 1/3 is wasted on errors and inefficiency. In fact, medical error is the third leading cause of death in the U.S. annually, taking roughly 250,000 lives per year, according to an estimate published in the *Journal of the American Medical Association.* This includes hospital-acquired infections, unnecessary surgeries, medication errors and medical malpractice.[113] And who gets admitted to the hospital? Of the top five reasons for hospital admission, *heart disease* accounts for three.[114]

To avoid meat is to avoid the diseases and the lengthy hospital stays that drain the household, the nation and the globe. Without these diseases (heart attacks, atherosclerosis, congestive heart failure) and the costs they incur, insurance premiums will go down, universal health coverage will be a reality, and we'll have less of a need for hospitals, because we'll be less sick.

III. By eating plants, you heal the world, starting with yourself.

9. Plant eaters are stronger, faster, leaner, and longer-lived than meat eaters.

Clinical studies show that those who do not eat meat have more strength and stamina, recover faster and live 5 to 10 years longer than meat-eaters.[115116]

10. A diet free of meat, eggs and diary is guilt-free, inexpensive and easy.

Buying, preparing and enjoying your own plant-centered cuisine provides you with health-sustaining nutrients and costs less than eating three fast food meals, which offer nothing but empty calories that promise to make you sick, tired and fat. Not only that, but nutrient for nutrient, fast food is several times more expensive than a home cooked vegan meal.

Let's compare 1 cup of boiled spinach to one McDonald's apple pie. Spinach has 30 calories, apple pie has 260 calories. To get the amount of vitamin C in spinach (200 percent of the daily value), you'd have to eat 5 apple pies, and in so doing consume 1,300 calories and 60 grams of fat. And no amount of apple pies could ever equal the quality of fiber, water and most vitamins and minerals present in **one leaf of spinach!**

Start by observing one meatless day per week, Monday perhaps. After a few such weeks, extend it through Tuesday. Work towards a flesh-free week. Cook for yourself and your family. Love your animal brothers. Be an American for the new Millennium. Heal the world, starting with yourself.

APPENDIX E: PARADIGM PLANS

Let's face it, food is a touchy subject. Many are wed to their dietary indiscretions and fiercely defend themselves if criticized, and still more eat whatever is served, not just out of laziness but from conformity and convention as well. Peer pressure is a bitch!

So how do you apply the Paradigm in a world where fast food, packaged, processed fare, nuts, oils, meats and grains are so ubiquitous? The best and easiest way is to make your own food. Eat as many meals in the home as you can, and for the times you do eat out, pack a lunch or bring along a snack as often as you can. In other words, prepare to be prepared. And as a wise man once said, *Judge not lest you be judged.*

Yet we all find ourselves at parties or at restaurants where less than ideal food is served, usually in superabundance. Here are some tips to staying sane and saving face at your next picnic, party or Papa John's.

- When dining out, stick to salads, soups and sides of veggies.
- Eat half a meal before going to the party, and once there fill up on the vegetable platter before moving to the cheese plate.
- Indulge if you must, but remember how you feel the next day. It may be less than Paradigm. Experience is, after all, the great reinforcer. If you don't like the way processed food makes you feel, you'll be less likely to eat it again.

- Stay the course. The more committed you are to your new dietstyle, the more successful you'll be at maintaining it. Enthusiasm is infectious, so you may gain some converts along the way.
- Spread the love. Spread the word. Heal the world!

ABOUT THE AUTHOR

Adam Dave, M.D. trained in family medicine at one of the nation's top teaching hospitals, where his focus was on weight management through lifestyle modification. Valedictorian and recipient of the Dean's Award for academic excellence, Dr. Dave has worked extensively in the field of nutritional medicine. With his simple, diet-centered approach he has helped many achieve greater health and fitness and improve vitality and appearance. Accomplished distance runner and triathlete, in his spare time Dr. Dave can be found writing novels and running the hills of Hollywood, barefoot – often at the same time.

NOTES

1   *Dietary Guidelines for Americans 2010*; U.S. Department of Agriculture; U.S. Department of Human Services

2   Distinguished by what? At one time or another, we have been all of these personalities.

3   Shintani TT, Hughes CK, Beckham S, et al. Obesity and cardiovascular risk intervention through the ad libitum feeding of traditional Hawaiian diet. *Am. J. Clin. Nutr.* 14 (1994): 491-496.

4   Schroder KE. Effects of fruit consumption on body mass index and weight loss in a sample of overweight and obese dieters enrolled in a weight-loss intervention trial. *Nutrition.* (2010 Jul-Aug): 727-34.

5   Poehlman ET, Arciero PJ, Melby CL, et al. Resting metabolic rate and postprandial thermogenesis in vegetarians and nonvegetarians. *Am. J. Clin. Nutr.* 48. (1988): 209-213.

6   Esselstyn CJ. Introduction: more than coronary artery disease. *Am J. Cardiol.* 82 (1998): 5T-9T.

7   Anderson JW. Dietary fiber in nutrition management of diabetes. *In:* G. Vahouny, V. and D. Kritchevsky (eds.), *Dietary Fiber: Basic and Clinical Aspects,* pp. 343-360. New York: Plenum Press, 1986.

8   Appleby PN, Davey GK, Key TJ. Hypertension and blood pressure among meat eaters, fish eaters, vegetarians and vegans in EPIC-Oxford. *Public Health Nutr.* 2002 Oct; 5(5): 645-54.

9   Orgeta RM, Requejo AM, Andres P, et al. Dietary intake and cognitive function in a group of elderly people. *Am J. Clin. Nutr.* 66 (1997): 803-809.

10   Singh P et al. Does low meat consumption increase life expectancy in humans? *Am. J. Clin. Nutr.* 78 (2003): 526S-532S.

11   Krieger E, Youngman LD, and Campbell TC. The modulation of afla-toxin induced preneoplastic lesions by dietary protein and voluntary exercise in Fischer 344 rats. *FASEB J.* 2 (1988): 3304 Abs.

12   Food and Agriculture Organization *Statistical Yearbook*, 2009.

13   www.usda.gov Agriculture Fact Book, 2001-2002

14   The average American buys 200 lbs of fresh fruits and vegetables each year, and over 600 lbs of animal products and grains, which on average have 5 times as many calories as produce, per lb. This results in an intake of high-fat animal protein and refined grains that exceeds fruit and vegetable con-sumption by a factor of ten.

15   Lorson, BA, et al. Correlates of fruit and vegetable intakes in US chil-dren. *Journal of the American Dietetic Association.* Volume 109, Issue 3; March 2009 .

16   www.choosemyplate.gov

17   Kochanek, Kenneth, et al. National Vital Statistics Report. Deaths: Preliminary Data for 2009. Volume 59, Number 4. March 16, 2011.

18   *Dietary Reference Intakes for Energy, Carbohydrate, Fiber, Fat, Fatty Acids, Cholesterol, Protein, and Amino Acids: Chapter 12- Physical Activity*, pg. 889; Insti-tute of Medicine; 2005.

19   USDA National Nutrient Database for Standard Reference, available at www.nal.usda.gov/fnic/foodcomp/search/

20   *Dietary Reference Intakes for Energy, Carbohydrate, Fiber, Fat, Fatty Acids, Cholesterol, Protein, and Amino Acids: Chapter 5- Energy*, pg. 114; Institute of Medicine; 2005.

21   Brody, Jane. Research lifts blame from many of the obese. *NY Times.* March 24, 1987.

22   Armstrong D, and Doll R. Environmental factors and cancer incidence and mortality in different countries, with special reference to dietary practices. *Int. J. Cancer.* 15 (1975): 617-631.

23   Carroll KK, Braden LM, Bell JA, et al. Fat and cancer. *Cancer.* 58 (1986): 1818-1825.

24   Thiébaut ACM, et al. Dietary fat and postmenopausal invasive breast cancer in the National Institutes of Health-AARP Diet and Health Study Cohort. *J Natl Cancer Inst.* 2007; 99: 451–62.

25   *Pathologic Basis of Disease*; Vinay Kumar, M.D.; 2005.

26   Simopoulos AP: Essential fatty acids in health and chronic disease. *Am J Clin Nutr.* 1999; 70(Suppl): 560S-569S.

27   Lawrence, Felicity. Omega-3, junk food and the link between violence and what we eat. *The Guardian.* October, 2006.

28   Esparza ML, Sasaki S, Kesteloot H: Nutrition, latitude, and multiple sclerosis morality: An ecologic study. *Am J Epidemiol.* 1995; 142: 733-777.

29   Morris, Martha, et al. Dietary fat and the risk of incident Alzheimer Disease. *Archives of Neurology.* 2003; 60: 194-200.

30   Kavanagh, K. Trans fat diet induces abdominal obesity and changes in insulin sensitivity in monkeys. *Obesity.* 2007 Jul; 15(7): 1675-84.

31   Hegsted, D. Minimum protein requirements of adults. *American Journal of Clinical Nutrition.* 21 (1968): 3520.

32   *The China Study*; T. Colin Campbell, Ph.D.; 2006.

33   *Nutritive Value of American Foods in Common Units*; USDA Agriculture Handbook No. 456.

34   Doi SQ, Rasaiah S, Tack I, et al. Low-protein diet suppresses serum insulin-like growth factor-1 and decelerates the progression of growth hor-Mone-induced glomerulosclerosis. *Am. J. Nephrol.* 21 (2001): 331-339.

35   Heaney RP, McCarron DA, Dawson-Hughes B, et al. Dietary changes favorably affect bone remodeling in older adults. *J. Am. Diet. Assoc.* 99 (1999): 1228-1233.

36   Allen NE, Appleby PN, Davey GK, et al. Hormones and diet: low insulin-like growth factor-I but normal bioavailable androgens in vegan men. *Brit. J. Cancer.* 83 (2000): 95-97.

37   *Biochemistry*; Pamela C. Champe, et al.; 2005.

38   Joint FAO/WHO/UNU Expert Consultation on Protein and Amino Acid Requirements in Human Nutrition (2002). Geneva, Switzerland

39   USDA National Nutrient Database for Standard Reference

40   *Healthy at 100: The Scientifically Proven Secrets of the World's Healthiest and Longest-lived Peoples*; John Robbins; 2006.

41   Andoh, A., et al. Role of dietary fiber and short-chain fatty acids in the colon. *Current Pharmaceutical Design.* 2003;9(4): 347-58.

42   *Dietary Reference Intakes for Energy, Carbohydrate, Fiber, Fat, Fatty Acids, Cholesterol, Protein, and Amino Acids (Macronutrients) (2005);* National Academy of Sciences, Institute of Medicine, Food and Nutrition Board.

43www.clemson.edu/extension/hgic/food/nutrition/nutrition/special_nee
ds/hgic4151.html

44   Bates, Graham P., et al. Sweat rate and sodium loss during workout in
the heat. *J Occup Med Toxicol.* 2008; 3: 4.

45   Linus Pauling Institute at Oregon State University: Micronutrient Information Center: Sodium (Chloride); Jane Higdon, Ph.D.; 2004.

46   www.nlm.nih.gov/medlineplus/ency/article/003887.htm

47   Gear, J.S.S., et al. Fibre and bowel transit times. *Br. J. Nutr.* (1981) **45**,
77.

48   *Oxygen Radical Absorbance Capacity of Selected Foods*; Nutrient Data Laboratory; 2007

49   Collens, W. Atherosclerotic Disease: An Anthropologic Theory. *Medical Counterpoint*, pg. 54, Dec 1969.

50   Roach, John. Cannibalism normal for early humans? *National Geographic
News.* April 2003.

51   Adapted with permission from Joel Fuhrman, M.D.

52   Please see *Eat for Health*, by Joel Fuhrman, M.D.

53   X. Wu et al. Lipophilic and hydrophilic antioxidant capacities of common foods in the United States. *Journal of Agricultural and Food Chemistry.* 52,
no. 12 (June 9, 2004): 4026-4037.

54   The only nutrient lacking is vitamin D, which your skin can synthesize
on exposure to the sun.

55   *Medical Microbiology & Immunology*; Warren Levinson, M.D., Ph.D.;
2004.

56 www.fda.gov/Food/FoodSafety/ProductSpecificInformation/Seafood/
ConsumerInformationAboutSeafood/ucm122607.htm

57   www.ncbi.nlm.nih.gov/pubmedhealth/PMH0001280/

58   www.glycemicindex.com

59   Hoyt, Garrett, et al. Dissociation of the glycaemic and insulinaemic
responses to whole and skimmed milk. *British Journal of Nutrition.* (2005), 93:
175-177.

60   www.cspinet.org/nah/05_06/grains.pdf

61   Slavin, Joan. Whole grains and human health. *Nutrition Research Reviews.*
(2004), 17, 000–000.

62 www.fda.gov/food/labelingnutrition/FoodAllergensLabeling/Guidance
ComplianceRegulatoryInformation/ucm106187.htm

63   www.aaemonline.org/gmopost.html

64   "The Truth about Herpes," from www.herpes.com.

65   *CDC Morbidity and Mortality Weekly Report, March 2010*

66   Griffith, RS, et al. Relation of arginine-lysine antagonism to herpes
simplex growth in tissue culture. *Chemotherapy.* 1981; 27(3): 209-13.

67   United States Department of Agriculture Fact Book, 2001-2002

68   Christian, Paul, et al. Effects of meal size and correction technique on
gastric emptying time: studies with two tracers and opposed detectors. *J Nucl
Med.* 21: 883-885,1980.

69   *Dietary Reference Intakes (DRIs): Recommended Dietary Allowances and Adequate Intakes, Vitamins;* Food and Nutrition Board, Institute of Medicine,
National Academies.

70   McDougall, John. Vitamin B12 deficiency: The meat-eater's last stand. *McDougall Newsletter.* Vol. 6, No. 11. November 2007.

71   Albert, M.J. Vitamin B12 synthesis by human intestinal bacteria. *Nature.* 1980 Feb 21; 283(5749): 781-2.

72   ods.od.nih.gov/factsheets/VitaminB12-HealthProfessional/

73   ods.od.nih.gov/factsheets/vitamind/

74   Milaneschi, Y., et al. Serum 25-hydroxyvitamin D and depressive symptoms in older women and men. *The Journal of Clinical Endocrinology and Metabolism.* July 2010.

75   Chai W. Effect of different cooking methods on vegetable oxalate content. *J. Agric. Food Chem.* 2005 April 20; 53(8): 3027-30.

76   Please see: *The Food Revolution;* John Robbins; 2010.

77   "The Price of Beef," WorldWatch, July/August 1994, p. 39.

78   Carus, Felicity. UN urges global move to meat and dairy free diet. Guardian.co.uk. Wednesday June 2 2010.

79   Please see: *The World's Healthiest Foods;* George Mateljan; 2007.

80   www.choosemyplate.gov

81   For more information, please see: *The World's Healthiest Foods;* George Mateljan; 2007.

82   Tofu is a chewy, cheese-like food made from soybeans. Though not a whole food, it may help you transition away from meat and cheese. Tofu makes a nice addition to both cooked vegetables and salads, as it acts like a sponge and soaks up any flavor. Freezing tofu gives it a meaty texture. Buy only organic varieties, and enjoy no more than a couple times per week. Keep in mind, however, that tofu is 50 percent fat and a concentrated source of omega-6 fatty acids. Besides, humans have only been eating tofu

since 200 B.C., less than the amount of time we've been eating grains, shorter even than we've consumed milk products *and only a fraction of a percent as long as the millions of years we've been consuming unprocessed plants!* One could argue that our digestion has not adapted, which could explain the *tofu bloat.*

83   *Pathologic Basis of Disease*; Vinay Kumar et al.; 2005.

84   USDA Database for the Oxygen Radical Absorbance Capacity (ORAC) of Selected Foods, Release 2

85   http://www.nhlbisupport.com/bmi/

86   Fisher, Irving, The Influence of Flesh Eating on Endurance, *Yale Medical Journal*, 13(5):205-221, 1907.

87   For a more accurate measurement of your frame size, please visit www.nlm.nih.gov/medlineplus/ency/imagepages/17182.htm

88   *Eat, Drink, and Be Healthy*; Walter Willett, M.D.; 2005.

89   www.acefitness.org/calculators/bodyfat-calculator.aspx

90   Please see: *The 80/10/10 Diet*; Dr. Douglas Graham; 2006.

91   The term *fun exercise* should not be a contradiction. Movement is as natural as breathing or laughing. Inactivity, on the other hand, is constipation. Not exactly fun.

92   Sadly, for many teens, TV, computers and video games have reduced movement to the twitch of a thumb.

93   From an economic perspective, of the two decisions, to avoid college and not to exercise, the latter could wind up costing more. There are many self-made millionaires without a college degree, but few sedentary folk enjoy vigor to a ripe old age; and medical bills, especially as a result of chronic diseases directly influenced by diet and exercise, are the number one cause of bankruptcy.

94   Factors involved in the freshman five include fast food, not enough exercise, and of course, cheap beer.

95   Making exercise a lifelong commitment maintains muscle mass and keeps the metabolism revved up.

96   Harder workouts can be performed less frequently, as high intensity training achieves the same results in shorter periods.

97   *Dietary Reference Intakes for Energy, Carbohydrate, Fiber, Fat, Fatty Acids, Cholesterol, Protein, and Amino Acids (Macronutrients) (2005)* National Academy of Sciences. Institute of Medicine. Food and Nutrition Board: Chapter 12 – Physical Activity

98   Please see: *Born to Run*; Christopher McDougall; 2009.

99   Please see: *Barefoot Running Step by Step*; Ken Bob Saxton and Roy M. Wallack; 2011.

100 To determine whether you have this condition and to easily correct it, please visit triggerpointworkbook.com/mortons.htm.

101 Please see: *The Trigger Point Therapy Workbook*; Claire Davies; 2004.

102 To calculate BMI: http://www.nhlbisupport.com/bmi/

103 To calculate BFP: http://www.healthstatus.com/calculate/body-fat-calculator-navy

104 ods.od.nih.gov/factsheets/vitaminb12/

105 McDougall, John. Vitamin B12 deficiency: The meat-eater's last stand. *McDougall Newsletter*. Vol. 6, No. 11. November 2007.

106 Suzuki, H. Serum vitamin B12 levels in young vegans who eat brown rice. *J Nutr Sci Vitaminol (Tokyo)*. 1995 Dec;41(6): 587-94.

107 *The China Study*; T. Colin Campbell, Ph.D.; 2006.

108 Please see: *Diet for a New America*; John Robbins; 1987.

109 Carus, Felicity. UN urges global move to meat and dairy free diet. Guardian.co.uk. Wednesday June 2 2010.

110 Walsh, Brian. Meat: Making global warming worse. Time Health. Wednesday, September 10, 2008.

111 Linares, M.B. et al. Cortisol and catecholamine levels in lambs: Effects of slaughter weight and type of stunning. *Livestock Science*. Volume 115, Issue 1, pg. 53-61, May 2008.

112 Young, E.A. et al. Cortisol and catecholamines in posttraumatic stress disorder: An epidemiologic community study. *Archives of General Psychiatry*. 2004 Apr; 61(4):394-401.

113 Allen, Marshall. First do no harm. *Washington Monthly*. March/April 2011.

114 Most Common Diagnoses and Procedures in U.S. Community Hospitals, 1996. Healthcare Cost and Utilization Project, Research Note. AHCPR Publications No. 99-0046. Rockville, MD. Agency for Healthcare Policy and Research, 1999.

115 Fisher, Irving. The influence of flesh eating on endurance. *Yale Medical Journal*, 13(5): 205-221, 1907.

116 Astrand, Per-Olaf, *Nutrition Today* 3: no2, 9-11, 1986.

13230505R00168

Made in the USA
Lexington, KY
20 January 2012